Acid Reflux Diet & Cookbook

FOR

DUMMIES®

A Wiley Brand

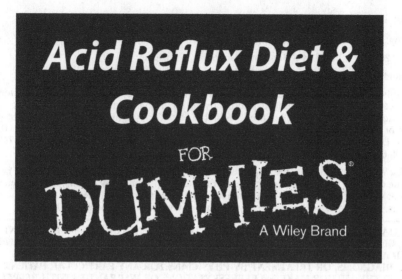

Acid Reflux Diet & Cookbook

FOR DUMMIES®

A Wiley Brand

by Dr. Patricia Raymond and
Michelle Beaver

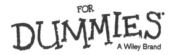

Acid Reflux Diet & Cookbook For Dummies®

Published by: **John Wiley & Sons, Inc.,** 111 River Street, Hoboken, NJ 07030-5774, www.wiley.com

Copyright © 2014 by John Wiley & Sons, Inc., Hoboken, New Jersey

Published simultaneously in Canada

For general information on our other products and services, please contact our Customer Care Department within the U.S. at 877-762-2974, outside the U.S. at 317-572-3993, or fax 317-572-4002. For technical support, please visit www.wiley.com/techsupport.

Wiley publishes in a variety of print and electronic formats and by print-on-demand. Some material included with standard print versions of this book may not be included in e-books or in print-on-demand. If this book refers to media such as a CD or DVD that is not included in the version you purchased, you may download this material at http://booksupport.wiley.com. For more information about Wiley products, visit www.wiley.com.

Library of Congress Control Number: 2014935507

ISBN 978-1-118-83919-5 (pbk); ISBN 978-1-118-83915-7 (ebk); ISBN 978-1-118-83914-0 (ebk)

Manufactured in the United States of America

SKY10025873_032421

Contents at a Glance

Recipes at a Glance

Main Courses

Desserts

Main Courses

Table of Contents

Introduction

. . . .

*A*cid reflux isn't fun. It isn't healthy, and it isn't something you want in your life. Even if your acid reflux is only a minor annoyance, you'd still like to get rid of it. *Acid Reflux Diet & Cookbook For Dummies* is one of the best tools you can use to curb your condition or get rid of it completely.

Other important resources: your doctor and determination. Your doctor can help you diagnose your acid reflux and monitor your symptoms and treatment. As for determination, you'll need that to follow your doctor's recommendations and the guidelines in this book. The diet and recommendations you'll find here aren't extremely difficult, but fortitude will come in handy anyway.

This book helps you understand what acid reflux is, what causes it, what the dangers are, and most important, how to reduce your symptoms or get rid of the condition all together.

About This Book

Change isn't easy, especially when that change involves diet and other alterations to your daily life. This book, however, makes change about as easy as it can be, by offering clear advice in an accessible format. You don't have to read this book from beginning to end. Consider it a reference manual, like an encyclopedia. You can look up the information that interests you the most. You can cherry-pick chapters by only reading those that are most applicable to you, or you can read all of them but out of order. And, of course, you can always be traditional and ready every chapter, in order.

Sidebars and anything marked by the Technical Stuff icon are skippable. Yes, these passages enhance the main sections, but the main sections will still make sense without the supplements.

In this book you may note that some web addresses break across two lines of text. If you're reading this in print and want to visit one of these web pages, simply type in the web address exactly as it's noted in the text, as though the line break doesn't exist. If you're reading this as an e-book, you've got it easy — just click the web address to be taken directly to the web page.

Finally, we follow a few basic conventions in the recipes that you should be aware of:

- ✔ Milk is whole unless otherwise specified.
- ✔ Eggs are large.
- ✔ Pepper is freshly ground black pepper unless otherwise specified.
- ✔ Butter is unsalted.
- ✔ Flour is all-purpose unless otherwise specified.
- ✔ Sugar is granulated unless otherwise noted.
- ✔ All herbs are fresh unless dried herbs are specified.
- ✔ All temperatures are in Fahrenheit. (Refer to the appendix for information about converting temperatures to Celsius.)
- ☻ We use the tomato icon to highlight vegetarian recipes in the Recipes in This Chapter lists, as well as in the Recipes in This Book.

Foolish Assumptions

We assume you're reading this book because you have acid reflux or because you care about someone who has acid reflux and you want to help. Either way, we know that you realize acid reflux is no bueno. This book doesn't waste time trying to convince you that acid reflux is annoying or painful — you already know that. You want to find out how to get rid of acid reflux, and how to do so as easily as possible.

Icons Used in This Book

We use icons to draw your attention to certain key points:

Text marked by the Tip icon is a quick-hit pointer that may or may not appear in the main text. If the tip is applicable to you, give it a try!

Anything marked by the Remember icon is a helpful bit of information to keep in mind, but it doesn't necessarily require action.

Beware! Text marked with the Warning icon tells you what not to mess with, and why.

 Some people like to hear the nitty-gritty details. The why behind the how and the how behind the why. Other people aren't as interested. If you usually like the subtext behind what you're reading, and you have the time to read it, check out anything marked with the Technical Stuff icon.

Beyond the Book

Check out a free Cheat Sheet at www.dummies.com/cheatsheet/ acidrefluxdiet for quick-hit resources not found in this book. The Cheat Sheet content is a handy reference that you can check out over and over online, print out, and/or refer to quickly and easily when you may not have your book handy.

In addition, www.dummies.com/extras/acidrefluxdiet contains related articles such as a guide to eating out and an exercise plan to reduce reflux.

Where to Go from Here

You've made an important decision on the acid reflux–reduction path: You bought this book. So, where do you go from here? That's up to you — you can read the chapters in whatever order suits you. If you already have a good understanding of reflux, you can skip to the recipes in Part III. Use the table of contents and index to find the subjects you're interested in right now.

However you want to use these chapters and regardless of the order you read them in, we wish you a successful and relatively easy transition toward a life with less acid reflux.

Part I
Getting Started with the Acid Reflux Diet

getting started

with

the Acid Reflux Diet

In this part . . .

- ✔ Diagnose acid reflux.
- ✔ Discover the dangers of acid reflux.
- ✔ Find over-the-counter medications for reflux.
- ✔ Identify your trigger foods.
- ✔ Talk with your doctor about your symptoms.

Chapter 1

Saying Goodbye to Reflux: Your Road to a Reflux-Free Lifestyle

A cid reflux is a common medical condition that affects millions of people around the globe. For some, reflux is a minor inconvenience, but others battle reflux daily. Your reflux may not require anything more than the occasional antacid. Or your fight with reflux could require daily medication, lifestyle changes, and even surgery. Regardless of where you fall on the spectrum, acid reflux has an impact.

The battle against reflux isn't always easy. Some days, the struggle may not seem worth the results, but in the long run, eliminating reflux is worth the effort. Not only will you be healthier and reduce your risk for serious medical complications associated with reflux, but you'll also just plain feel better.

What Acid Reflux Is, and Why It's Bad

Acid reflux is a digestive disorder that affects millions of people worldwide. Unlike many diseases or disorders, it doesn't discriminate. It affects all ages, races, ethnicities, and genders equally. Just because your family doesn't have a history of reflux doesn't mean you won't get reflux. Likewise, all your siblings having the condition doesn't mean you'll get it. Reflux also varies significantly in severity and frequency. Regardless of who it affects or how severe it gets, reflux is the result of a malfunctioning digestive system.

Depending on your symptoms, your doctor may diagnose you with acid reflux or gastroesophageal reflux disease (GERD). The root problem is the same for both of these conditions; it's the severity and frequency that separates the two. Patients who suffer heartburn or other reflux symptoms two or more times a week will usually be diagnosed with GERD. While GERD is usually the more serious condition, both acid reflux and GERD can lead to long-term health consequences.

The main culprit in all acid-reflux cases is the lower esophageal sphincter (LES), a small ring of muscles that connects the esophagus and the stomach. The esophagus is the tube that extends from the mouth to the stomach. This tube carries anything you eat or drink into the stomach. When your LES is working correctly, it functions as a one-way valve, allowing food and fluids to pass into the stomach while blocking any stomach contents from coming back up.

If you have acid reflux or GERD, your LES is malfunctioning. Instead of blocking the stomach's contents, the contents are allowed to travel back up into the esophagus. Because stomach acid is highly corrosive, it doesn't take much to cause discomfort and do some damage. Depending on how severe your reflux is, acid can make it all the way up to the larynx, throat, and mouth. In some cases that fiery fury can even make it into the lungs.

The reason why the LES malfunctions varies from person to person. In some cases, the LES may not close off completely after food or fluid passes through. Because the stomach works like a washing machine on spin cycle when digesting, a partially open LES means churning stomach acid can easily whirl out of the stomach. In other cases, your LES may simply open and close on its own, allowing your stomach's contents to escape. Sometimes the factor is lifestyle or weight; for other people, it's anatomy. Regardless of the root cause, how often and how severely your LES malfunctions will have a tremendous impact on how serious your acid reflux turns out to be.

Several symptoms are associated with acid reflux. The most common symptom is heartburn. Heartburn is so common that many people mistakenly refer to heartburn and acid reflux as the same thing. Heartburn is the burning sensation that results from stomach acid surging into the esophagus. Acid reflux is the condition that allows acid to make it into the esophagus. Although the pain associated with heartburn can be severe — so severe that it's sometimes mistaken for a heart attack — it's usually not a serious medical condition.

Some of the other relatively innocuous symptoms of acid reflux include gas, burping, bloating, regurgitation, and nausea. Although these symptoms may not seem serious, dealing with them on a regular basis can hamper your life.

Reflux is also linked with several serious, life-threatening medical conditions. One of the more serious conditions associated with reflux is *esophageal stricture* (a narrowing of the esophagus), which can make it difficult to swallow and often requires surgery to correct. Even more serious is *Barrett's esophagus,* a mutation of the cells lining the esophagus; this condition can be a precursor to esophageal cancer. No thank you.

It's not just the possible medical complications that make treating reflux or GERD worthwhile. Reflux affects life in so many other ways as well. It affects mood and emotions and sleep. When you're constantly dealing with discomfort or having to worry if your next meal is going to lead to hours of pain, it's hard to live in the moment. When you can't get a good night's sleep because of reflux, it makes each day that much longer and harder to get through. Add the constant stress your body is under from having to repair the physical damage that results from reflux, and it's a recipe for misery. So, even if you don't think your reflux is too bad, go ahead and take the challenge of reducing your reflux, and see how much better you feel.

Revamping Diet and Lifestyle

For some people, diet and lifestyle changes are easy. For you, it might be a long journey that can leave you feeling like you're sacrificing just as much as you're gaining. But keep with it! When your reflux is under control, all the effort will have been worth it. The other big advantage of treating reflux with lifestyle and dietary changes is monetary. Medication or surgery can be extremely expensive, but lifestyle and dietary changes are inexpensive.

Even just a few tweaks to diet can sometimes make a world of difference for your reflux. And diet is often one of the primary triggers for reflux symptoms like heartburn. You can probably name at least one meal that you know spells trouble for your reflux. But figuring out what exactly it is about that meal that's causing the flare-up can be difficult. Is it the ingredients, the sauce, the spices, or even how it's prepared?

Several foods seem to universally affect people's acid reflux and GERD negatively:

  ✔ **High-fat foods:** High-fat foods can sit in the stomach longer, which stimulates the body to produce more stomach acid. The more stomach acid you have spinning around in your stomach, the more likely some of it will enter the esophagus. Fatty and greasy foods cause the LES to relax. So, while there's more stomach acid splashing around for a longer period of time, there's also a weakened LES trying to keep your stomach contents where they belong. That's asking a lot of your body.

✔ **Spicy foods:** These foods can be troublesome for patients with reflux and GERD. They don't affect everyone as universally as high-fat foods, but it's not uncommon for patients to complain of severe heartburn after an extra spicy or flavorful meal.

✔ **Meals with lots of ingredients:** Some dietitians believe that complicated meals with lots of ingredients can be difficult to digest. Meals like these sit in the stomach longer, which can give your reflux an extended period of time to strike.

✔ **Highly acidic foods:** Even if they don't actually cause reflux, highly acidic foods can increase the pain and damage done to an already inflamed and irritated esophagus and throat.

✔ **Processed foods:** Staying away from processed foods is a good idea. Some dietitians believe that the body has to work harder to break down processed foods. Just like fatty foods, this may mean more gastric acid and a longer digestion period — prime reflux conditions. The longer food remains in the stomach, the more gastric acid is stimulated, and that longer timeframe presents more opportunities for gastric contents to regurgitate up the esophagus. Foods that are hard to mechanically digest, or grind up in the stomach, hang out longer.

It turns out when and how much you eat can have just as much of an impact on your reflux as what you eat. Most people are used to the traditional three daily meals with dinner being the largest. Although this may be tradition, it spells trouble for reflux. Eating only three meals a day (instead of smaller, more frequent meals) makes you more likely to overindulge at any given meal. Even if you don't overindulge, the meals are probably bigger than they'd be if you ate five meals a day. When you eat a large meal, it forces your stomach to stretch out. This puts more pressure on the LES, increasing the likelihood that it will fail and some stomach acid will escape. This is why binge eating is never a good idea, especially for people with reflux or GERD.

Instead of the traditional three large meals, try switching to five smaller meals. This will keep you from getting hungry and will put less stress on your stomach and LES. You should also try to eat your largest meal of the day for breakfast and keep your dinner relatively small. You'll have more energy during the day and your body won't be processing food at night. Because heartburn and reflux are usually worse at night, eating a smaller meal means quicker digestion and less opportunity for reflux. You should also wait at least two or three hours before lying down after a meal. The more time you give your body to digest before going to sleep, the lower the chance for heartburn.

By far the most important component in most people's battle with reflux is weight. While the exact reason or mechanism that excess weight causes or triggers reflux isn't known, researchers suspect that extra weight stresses the digestive system. Excess weight, especially abdominal weight, increases the amount of pressure on the stomach, which makes it possible for the stomach's contents to be pushed into the esophagus. Studies have also found that excess fat can impair the body's ability to empty the stomach quickly. The longer food sits, the more opportunity reflux has to strike.

Losing even a few pounds may be all you need to do in order to reduce or even eliminate reflux from your life completely. In fact, several studies have found that weight loss can be the most effective method of treatment for both acid reflux and GERD. And you don't even have to be very overweight for weight to play a factor. Research has shown that even for patients within their proper body mass index (BMI), the loss of a few pounds had significant impact on their reflux. A recent study of women found that losing weight reduced their risk for heartburn up to 40 percent.

To find your BMI, go to www.nhlbi.nih.gov/guidelines/obesity/BMI/bmicalc.htm. You just enter your height and weight, and you find your BMI.

Losing weight with reflux isn't just about working out. In fact, some types of workouts exacerbate reflux. Physicians usually recommend avoiding high-impact workouts, such as running. You'll also want to avoid exercises that increase the pressure on your stomach, such as crunches. Instead, try going hiking or walking. Low-impact exercise routines will still get those endorphins going and calories burning, without adding stress to the LES. Couple your workout with a balanced meal plan, and you'll be well on your way to dropping a few pounds and giving acid reflux the boot.

Habits like smoking tobacco, drinking alcohol, or consuming large amounts of caffeine can also affect reflux or GERD. Often these are the hardest habits for people to kick, because many of these items are stimulants with addictive qualities. Stop drinking caffeine out of the blue, and you're bound to experience headaches. Stop cigarettes cold turkey, and you're going to have a few miserable weeks ahead of you.

Tobacco use, no matter what type, has been linked to acid reflux and GERD. Studies have shown that tobacco inhibits saliva production. That's bad, because saliva plays a critical role in the digestion process. Saliva helps break down food and it also clears out food or acid from the esophagus. Less saliva means less efficient digestion. Tobacco also increases stomach acid production. This means there's more acid available to cause damage during a bout of reflux. On top of that, tobacco smoke can irritate an already sore esophagus, throat, and lungs.

Caffeine is another type of stimulant that can affect reflux. The good news for caffeine lovers is that it's usually overconsumption of caffeine that's the problem. For most people, one or two cups of coffee in a day isn't going to have a tremendous impact on their reflux. But putting down cup after cup throughout the day can spell problems.

The scientific community continues to waffle on the association between caffeinated coffee and reflux. A recent 2014 *meta-analysis* (a pooling together of 15 separate studies to try to come to a statistically significant conclusion) found "no significant association between coffee intake and GERD." However, other studies demonstrate that caffeine hurts the performance of the LES. To make it even more unclear to coffee lovers, darker roasts, which contain higher concentrations of chemicals such as N-methylpyridinium (which is produced by roasting the beans) have been shown to stimulate less gastric acid secretion than their lighter-roasted brethren, even with the same caffeine content. Confusing, right?

Bottom line: It's up to you and your body. If your light-roast, fully caffeinated coffee causes chest burning, perhaps consider a dark-roasted decaffeinated brew, or no coffee at all.

Another type of beverage to monitor: soda. Not only do many sodas contain caffeine, but the carbonic acid itself and carbonation can cause gas and bloating, symptoms that can intensify reflux.

Finally, your doctor will probably want to examine how much alcohol you consume. Any form of alcohol can be a nuisance for reflux. For instance, high-proof liquors interfere with the clearing of acid from the esophagus, especially when the subject is lying down. Basically, the high-proof alcohol slows down the esophageal muscles and the acid sits in the esophagus after it spurts up from the stomach. This means any corrosive acid that has managed to make it into the esophagus will have more time to damage your esophageal lining, making it more likely that you'll develop complications like esophageal strictures or even Barrett's esophagus.

Interestingly, while studies have found that alcohol can worsen reflux, they've also found that cutting back doesn't necessarily have a significant impact on reducing reflux. But that doesn't mean it's not worth the effort. Reducing alcohol may not cure your reflux, but continuing to consume it can certainly make reflux worse.

Cooking Your Way to Less Reflux

One way you can take control over your battle with acid reflux is to begin cooking your meals at home. We all know how easy it is to just grab a quick bite from a restaurant after work or between picking up the kids at school and dropping them off at basketball practice. However, taking the extra time to prepare meals at home may be worth the effort. If you need to eat out, follow the guidelines in Chapter 15.

Different foods affect people in different ways. Garlic may not bother you, but tomato sauce may be your kryptonite. So, part of the battle will be paying attention to what specific foods trigger your reflux. If you notice you get bad heartburn every time you eat an orange, it's a pretty good sign that you should avoid that food. In general, you should avoid foods that contain tomatoes, citrus, chocolate, and mint. Try to avoid cooking meals that use these particular ingredients, or figure out a substitute for the problem ingredient.

Another key is trying to make lighter, lower-fat meals. One easy way to do this is to bake or steam your food instead of frying or sautéing it. It's a quick and easy way to cut some of the fat from your meal and make it easier for your body to digest. Also try substituting lowfat yogurt for cream. Small recipe tweaks like that can go a long way in your fight against reflux. Cutting back on your meat portions and increasing your vegetable servings can also be helpful. Meats, especially those high in fat, take longer to empty from your stomach, which can be a problem for reflux sufferers. Finally, include as many whole grains in your diet as possible (as long as you don't have an allergy). Whole grains are filling and nutritious.

Drinking water with or right after your meal can also be a good way to reduce reflux symptoms, especially heartburn. Water will help flush stomach acid or food out of your esophagus and back down into your stomach. On top of that, water can dilute any acid trapped in the esophagus. The more diluted acid is, the less damage it can do. Although water can be helpful, you should avoid drinking carbonated water. Carbonated water can increase the pressure inside the stomach which can make the LES malfunction.

Just as there are foods you should avoid because they can trigger reflux, there are also foods that can reduce your risk for reflux. Oatmeal is always a good choice. Not only is it healthy in general, but it's also a lowfat, high-fiber meal that can help soothe the stomach. Ginger is another great ingredient for people with reflux. It has anti-inflammatory qualities and is often used to treat digestive and gastrointestinal issues, such as reflux. According to some dietitians, fruits like bananas and melons are often tolerated well by people who suffer from reflux.

In a small percentage of patients, bananas and melons can actually make reflux worse. Generally, you should look for fruits with a higher pH and avoid acidic fruits like oranges or lemons.

Try to incorporate as many greens and roots into your diet as possible. Vegetables like cauliflower, broccoli, asparagus, and green beans are all very nutritious and won't contribute to your reflux or GERD, unless you deep-fry them. Fennel can be another great food in the battle against reflux. Studies have shown that it helps to soothe the stomach while improving its function and efficiency. Slice it thin and add it to a salad or a chicken dish for a quick, healthy, heartburn-free meal. And don't be afraid of eating a few complex carbohydrates, such as brown rice. They'll give you fiber and energy and won't cause problems for your reflux.

The other thing you'll want to pay attention to is your choice of protein. Instead of eating high-fat meats, including most red meats, try switching over to leaner choices like chicken or turkey. Sometimes just switching to a leaner meat can be all it takes to reduce raging reflux to a manageable condition. The good thing about lean meats is that you can cook them in a variety of ways to keep from getting bored with the same meal day-in and day-out. Go ahead and bake, broil, grill, or sauté your poultry, but be sure to remove the skin because it's high in fat. Also, try incorporating more fish and seafood into your diet. Most types of fish are great lowfat choices.

Tackling Special Situations

A wide variety of special circumstances can influence a treatment plan for acid reflux and GERD. Some of the more common groups — such as pregnant women, kids, and the elderly — are covered in Chapter 16. But there are other unique situations that can affect your treatment, too.

One special case is acid reflux caused by a *hiatal hernia* (a condition in which a small section of the stomach gets pushed up into a hole in the diaphragm). Smaller hernias probably won't cause many noticeable symptoms; however, a larger hernia can cause food and stomach acid to get trapped in the esophagus, causing severe reflux and discomfort. In most cases, doctors may have to do some procedures (such as an upper endoscopy, esophageal pH test, or esophageal manometry) to verify if the hiatal hernia is the cause of the reflux. When your doctor has determined the cause, he'll map out a treatment plan.

There are a variety of treatments for hiatal hernias depending on the specifics of your condition. In some cases, the doctor may prescribe over-the-counter antacids or even prescription acid reflux medication. Treatment will also usually require you to adjust eating and sleeping schedules. It'll be important for you to eat several small meals a day — try to minimize the amount of food you eat at any one time. This will help reduce the likelihood that your reflux or GERD will flare up. You'll also want to avoid lying down for at least three hours after eating or drinking. In some cases, your doctor will recommend surgery to correct the problem. It's usually a laparoscopic procedure with a recovery time between five and ten days.

Treating your reflux or GERD while combating an ulcer is another special situation. For patients with both reflux and ulcers, the pain can be excruciating. Reflux symptoms tend to manifest in the upper chest, but ulcer pain usually falls between the sternum and navel. If you have a bad case of both, you could experience pain and discomfort in your whole chest and abdomen.

If your doctor determines that your ulcer has been caused by a bacteria living in the mucous coating your stomach *(Helicobacter pylori),* he'll treat the bacteria with strong antacid medications and antibiotics for 7 to 14 days. Successful treatment of *H. pylori* usually means that the recovered stomach lining then secretes even more acid, making your reflux symptoms worse, at least temporarily. After the *H. pylori* has been cleared, you may need lifelong antacid medication to manage the reflux.

Even generally innocuous over-the-counter medications like aspirin have been known to cause reflux flare-ups. Other medications that have been routinely linked to reflux and GERD include, antibiotics, steroids, antihistamines, heart medications, osteoporosis medications, chemotherapy drugs, pain medications, and even potassium and iron supplements.

Talk openly with your doctor and pharmacist about your reflux symptoms. It's a good idea to get all your medications through the same pharmacist so she can check for any drug interactions. The pharmacist may also be able to find a comparable medication that won't impact your reflux. And don't be afraid to try some of the usual remedies for reflux, such as a nice ginger tea or other stomach soothers.

Chapter 2

The Lowdown on Acid Reflux

In This Chapter

▶ Understanding the digestive process

▶ Identifying who develops acid reflux

▶ Seeing how acid reflux is diagnosed

*H*aving acid reflux gives you a front-row seat to understanding it. You know what acid reflux feels like, and you know that you don't like it. However, that obnoxious bile doesn't come with information about how to prevent it, what causes it, and how to diagnose it. The first step to beating reflux is to learn more about the condition.

Acid Reflux 101

Acid reflux is a remarkably common condition that affects millions of people worldwide. In the United States, more than 50 percent of people suffer occasionally from heartburn (one of the primary symptoms of acid reflux). And that's just the occasional bout. Nearly 30 percent of Americans suffer from acid reflux chronically.

Severity and frequency varies significantly from one person to the next. You may experience acid reflux once a month, but another person may have reflux daily and to a debilitating degree.

For some people, reflux is a long-term issue that they'll have to deal with for the rest of their lives, despite making changes. Others find that lifestyle changes and/or medication and surgery can eliminate their symptoms. Either way, heartburn can have a dramatic impact on a person's life.

Whether you suffer from reflux on a daily basis or only once a year, understanding acid reflux is important.

Heartburn versus acid reflux

When most people think about acid reflux, they immediately think of heartburn and use the words interchangeably. Although reflux and heartburn are related, they're not the same thing.

Heartburn is actually just a symptom of acid reflux. *Heartburn* is an uncomfortable or painful burning sensation in the chest that usually occurs after a meal. Just how much it hurts varies not only from person to person, but also from instance to instance. It can range from a mild irritation to an intense, searing pain.

Here's the easiest way to remember the difference between heartburn and acid reflux: Heartburn is the sensation, while acid reflux is the movement or action that *causes* the sensation.

The term *heartburn* can be somewhat misleading. First, heartburn has nothing to do with the heart; it's actually related to the digestive system, specifically the esophagus. Second, heartburn doesn't necessarily burn; it can be a general pain or a feeling of tightness in the chest. Many patients have rushed to the hospital thinking they were having a heart attack, only to find out it was actually an acute case of heartburn. These people have a hard time believing that a feeling that strong can "just" be heartburn.

If you think you're having a heart attack, take it very seriously and call 911 immediately. Symptoms of a heart attack can be subtle at first. Don't try to "tough it out." One symptom of heart attack is chest discomfort or pain. This may feel like pressure, fullness, or squeezing in the middle of your chest. The discomfort or pain may come and go. Other symptoms include body pain, anxiety, stomach illness, lightheadedness, sweating, and shortness of breath. Bottom line: Assume the symptoms you're experiencing may be heart-related until a physician has ruled it out.

Most people will experience at least one case of heartburn in their lifetimes. Lucky for them, occasional heartburn usually isn't anything to worry about and often can be cleared up with an antacid.

If you experience heartburn on a regular basis, you probably have acid reflux. Just like heartburn, acid reflux varies significantly in severity and frequency. It can be a daily problem that impacts your everyday life, or it can be a mild, occasional nuisance with little to no impact on your activities.

Severe, long-term cases of heartburn can lead to a diagnosis of gastroesophageal reflux disease (GERD). The condition is about as pleasant as the term. Go ahead and say it, "GERD." Rhymes with *turd.* Usually patients with GERD suffer from heartburn or other reflux symptoms at least twice a week. If you find that you're suffering from reflux on a regular basis, go to your doctor. Untreated reflux can develop into GERD, which can lead to more serious, long-term health issues.

What acid reflux does

Acid reflux is a digestive disorder that involves the esophagus and stomach. When you eat or drink, the contents travel down your esophagus and into your stomach. At the entrance to your stomach is a ring of muscle called the *lower esophageal sphincter* (LES). The LES is essentially a valve for the stomach. It relaxes to allow food or fluid to pass into the stomach and then tightens to prevent stomach contents from escaping up the esophagus.

When you have acid reflux, that usually means your LES is not functioning properly. When the LES is functioning normally, it closes after food or fluid passes. For people with acid reflux, this normal function is prevented. In some cases, this is a result of the muscles being weakened. In other cases, it's because of changes in abdominal pressure, especially in the stomach. Other times, the LES malfunctions and begins opening and closing itself. Regardless of the cause, the malfunction allows for your stomach contents, including stomach acid, to flow back into the esophagus.

The esophagus is above the stomach, so from a gravitational standpoint, it doesn't seem logical, even with a malfunctioning LES, that anything from the stomach would move back up. This just goes to show the power of what's going on in the stomach. The stomach functions like a washing machine — it's powerful. That's why you hear so much noise if you've ever had your ear near someone's stomach after a meal. When you combine churning stomach acid with a malfunctioning LES, a little reflux is inevitable, despite gravity.

A symptom of acid reflux, besides heartburn, is *dyspepsia* (stomach discomfort, usually of the upper abdomen). Heartburn can also create a feeling of fullness or bloating, burping, and nausea, usually after eating. This can lead to regurgitation, which is another common acid reflux symptom. Regurgitation occurs when the stomach's contents, including stomach acid, back up into the throat or mouth. Often, this results in a sour or bitter taste. In severe cases, regurgitation will cause vomiting.

Although regurgitation is the most common symptom, several other symptoms could be due to acid reflux. These include

- ✔ Asthma
- ✔ Chest pain
- ✔ Cough

✔ Dental erosion

✔ Difficulty swallowing

✔ Excess saliva

✔ Hoarseness

✔ Sore throat

What causes acid reflux

The exact cause of reflux can be difficult to pin down, but doctors and researchers do know that reflux happens most often after a large meal. Overeating can put extra pressure on the LES, making it more likely to fail. Also, bending over or lying down after a meal can cause or worsen a bout of reflux.

Some other factors are beyond your control. For instance, one contributor to acid reflux for some people is a hiatal hernia, which can occur at any age. A *hiatal hernia* happens when the upper part of the stomach and the LES are pushed above the diaphragm. The diaphragm is a muscular sheet under the lungs. It separates the stomach from the chest and allows you to inhale and exhale. Under normal circumstances, the diaphragm wraps around the lower end of the esophagus and also helps keep stomach acid out of the esophagus. However, when you have a hiatal hernia, the opening in the diaphragm is not as snug as it should be, so it's not helping the LES to remain closed and leads to reflux.

Pregnancy can also cause acid reflux (see "Pregnant women," later in this chapter, for more information). Happy day, though: That reflux usually disappears when the child is born.

Weight has also been shown to be a significant factor in many cases of reflux. Being overweight, specifically increased *abdominal girth* (also known as a big belly) increases the amount of pressure put on the abdominal organs, which in turn means more stress on the LES. Even if you aren't overweight by much, a few extra pounds can be all it takes to trigger acid reflux. The good news is that this works in reverse as well. Dropping a few extra pounds may mean no more reflux.

What and how you eat can also be a significant factor in reflux. Large meals force the stomach to expand more than it wants to, which puts too much pressure on the LES. The more pressure you put on the LES, the more likely it is to fail. And it's not just how much you eat that can give you reflux, it's also what you eat. The most common foods and drinks that have been linked with acid reflux include

- ✔ Alcohol
- ✔ Caffeinated beverages (*Note:* Caffeine doesn't bother everyone, but it may bother you. More on this controversial topic later.)
- ✔ Chocolate
- ✔ Citrus
- ✔ Coffee
- ✔ Fatty or fried foods
- ✔ Garlic
- ✔ Onions
- ✔ Spicy foods
- ✔ Tomatoes

Other personal habits can cause acid reflux as well. One significant example: smoking. Smoking briefly reduces the pressure of the LES while you've actively got a lit one in your mouth, in addition it chronically reduces saliva production and increases acid secretion in the stomach. All these factors can play a role in triggering heartburn and reflux. And that smoker's cough pushes acid up the esophagus as well. All additional reasons to work on that smoking cessation!

Some medications, whether they're prescribed or over the counter, can also result in acid reflux. This is why it's important to list all your medications when you discuss acid reflux with your doctor. Not knowing what's causing your reflux can make it difficult to figure out the best possible treatment.

How acid reflux can affect your life

Acid reflux can have a tremendous impact on a person's life. It can mean not eating certain foods or drinking certain drinks and not resting how or when you want to. It can mean you'll have to make difficult lifestyle changes, such as losing weight or quitting smoking. In some cases, it can also mean that you'll have to go on medication or have surgery. Reflux can even affect your personal relationships, if it makes you grouchy or prevents you from having the same sleep schedule as your partner.

Over the long term, chronic acid reflux and GERD can lead to serious health issues. For instance, GERD can increase the odds that you'll develop asthma. This is thought to occur when the nerves of the esophagus lining are irritated, causing contraction and narrowing of the muscles in the airway passages.

In the burning heart: Acid reflux and relationships

It's not just physical health that can be impacted by acid reflux; relationships can suffer, too. One man — we'll call him Jim — attributes the breakdown of his marriage to his acid reflux. A high-level manager in his company, Jim had been married for three years when he started to experience heartburn on an increasingly frequent basis. Instead of going to the doctor, he tried to self-medicate with antacids, which unfortunately did very little to alleviate his suffering.

At first, Jim admits, it was only a minor inconvenience. But as his symptoms began to get more intense and frequent, he started to have difficulty sleeping. It got to the point where three or four nights a week, he wasn't able to get more than a couple hours of rest. The lack of sleep combined with the severity of his symptoms caused him to become moody and impatient. And you guessed it, Jim's wife was the most frequent target of his outbursts. It got so bad that she decided she needed a break and moved into a local hotel.

Jim's wife leaving was the wake-up call he needed. Instead of trying to ignore his symptoms and, as he put it, "deal with the pain like a man," he finally made an appointment to see his doctor. It turned out that a combination of his weight, diet, smoking, and work stress was triggering his acid reflux. A few months of hard work later, his reflux symptoms were under control and more important, his wife was right back by his side.

The moral of the story here is that reflux can impact your life in a wide variety of ways. It isn't just the physical pain and potentially long-term damage reflux can do to your health. It's also the damage it can have on your personal relationships and your career.

And it isn't just breathing that can be affected by reflux. Long-term exposure to stomach acid can cause damage and scarring along the inside of your esophagus, larynx, and lungs. Long-term damage to the esophagus can make it difficult to swallow and make heartburn all the more painful. It also makes you more likely to develop Barrett's esophagus.

Barrett's esophagus occurs when the cells inside your esophagus mutate. These mutated cells are considered precancerous, and without treatment they can turn cancerous. Approximately 10 percent of patients with GERD end up with a diagnosis of Barrett's. So, take your acid reflux symptoms seriously, because over time, they can turn into a matter of life and death.

Who Gets Acid Reflux

Anyone can get acid reflux or suffer the occasional bout of heartburn. If you have a stomach and an esophagus, it could happen to you. More than 60 million people experience heartburn or other reflux symptoms at least once a month in the United States alone. Even more startling is that about 30 percent of U.S. residents have *chronic* acid reflux or GERD. But what does the average person who experiences reflux look like? In this section, we paint a picture for you.

Your average Jane and Joe

Most people who suffer acid reflux experience symptoms once or twice a month. In contrast, those with GERD can experience symptoms anywhere from twice a week to several times a day. That said, there are some factors that can increase your risk of experiencing the occasional case of heartburn.

Often, the development of acid reflux can be linked to personal habits. The first is weight. As mentioned earlier in this chapter, even a small amount of excess weight can trigger reflux. Likewise, eating a big meal can be a catalyst for discomfort. What you choose to eat and drink can impact reflux. Bad habits, such as smoking and drinking, often contribute to the chances you'll develop acid reflux. However, sometimes the factors that lead to reflux have little to do with personal choices.

Some people develop acid reflux because of physical problems. As mentioned, a hiatal hernia can be a gateway to reflux. Other people who have acid reflux get it because they were born with or developed a malformed or dysfunctional LES. Other people who have acid reflux got the condition because they developed abnormal esophageal contractions.

It doesn't matter if you are old or young, black or white, American or Chinese, anyone can develop acid reflux or GERD. It affects people at all economic levels and in all types of professions. And unlike many diseases, there is usually no genetic component. Your parents or siblings having acid reflux makes you no more likely to develop acid reflux than anyone else.

Pregnant women

It's common for women to experience their first bout of acid reflux during pregnancy. In fact, 50 percent of women develop some form of acid reflux during their pregnancy. The two most common acid-reflux symptoms during pregnancy are a burning sensation in the chest or throat and nausea. Most women report that their acid reflux is worst during the second and third trimesters.

There are two primary culprits when it comes to pregnancy and acid reflux:

- ✔ **Hormones:** When a woman becomes pregnant, she begins to produce more of a hormone called *progesterone*. Progesterone has been shown to slow the digestion process. The longer digestion occurs, the greater the chance that some stomach acid will splash into the esophagus. Some other pregnancy-related hormones have also been shown to weaken the LES, increasing the chances of a reflux flare up.

✔ **The baby itself:** As the baby takes up more and more real estate in the uterus, it pushes harder on the stomach. This upward force can push stomach acid into the esophagus. Combine a slowed digestion process with a growing baby, and it's easy to see why acid reflux may flare.

There are several things pregnant women can do to decrease the severity and frequency of acid reflux attacks, without harming their babies:

✔ **Eat five or six small meals per day instead of three large daily meals.** Larger meals take longer to digest and force the stomach to expand further. This makes it more likely that you'll experience reflux, especially with your digestion slowed by hormones.

✔ **Drink less with meals.** Drinking too much with your meal can slow digestion, and poor digestion can contribute to acid reflux.

✔ **Eat slowly.** Eating slowly will help you eat the right amount of food. It takes the brain about 20 minutes to realize that the stomach is full. If you wolf down your food, you'll have eaten way too much by the time that 20-minute marker rolls around and says you're full. Also, eating slowly means you chew more and are more relaxed. When you're relaxed and chew well, you'll digest your food better, and this will make acid reflux less likely.

✔ **Avoid lying down immediately after eating.** In general, you should wait at least two hours after a meal before lying down. When you do lie down, prop up your upper body slightly by placing pillows underneath your shoulders and down to your hips. This will help stop stomach acid from splashing into the esophagus. Try to not just lift your chest, because "crimping" yourself in the middle increases the abdominal pressure that worsens GERD.

✔ **Check with your doctor about over-the-counter antacids and heartburn relievers.** Some of these medications are safe to take during pregnancy. Most women find that liquid medication (which coats the esophageal lining) is the most effective remedy.

Usually pregnancy-related reflux can be diagnosed based on symptoms alone. It's rare that a doctor will want to do invasive testing to verify an acid-reflux diagnosis for a pregnant woman.

Your acid reflux likely won't impact your baby, so don't believe that old wives' tale that your baby will be born with heartburn as a result of your reflux.

Children

Children can experience acid reflux just like adults. Most children who get acid reflux experience their symptoms shortly after eating. Playing energetically (jumping, running) after meals and lying down after meals also makes reflux symptoms more likely and oftentimes more severe.

Unlike adults, the symptoms children experience as a result of their acid reflux often vary based on age. The most common symptoms for preschool-age children include weight loss, a lack of interest in food, regurgitation or vomiting, and in rare cases, wheezing. The wheezing is much more common in children who have been diagnosed with asthma. Children who can't talk yet will sometimes indicate their discomfort by pounding their chests.

Older children and adolescents can experience many of the same symptoms as their younger counterparts, and a wider range of symptoms. Older children are more likely to experience pain or burning in their upper chest (heartburn). They'll often complain that it's difficult to swallow or that they feel like food gets stuck in their throats. Complaints of nausea and vomiting are common, too. These children are more likely to awaken at night with abdominal pain or nausea.

If your child is experiencing any of these symptoms, talk with the child's doctor before beginning any treatment plan. Because there are several other medical issues that have reflux-like symptoms, confirming that it is, in fact, reflux is important. If the child doesn't have other medical problems as a result of reflux, doctors will usually recommend lifestyle changes. These changes include altering dietary habits, avoiding certain foods, losing weight, raising the head of the bed, and limiting exposure to cigarette smoke. The doctor may also recommend some acid reflux medications.

Children with complications as a result of their acid reflux often require additional medical testing. For instance, children who complain of difficulty or pain when swallowing may need an upper endoscopy test. If the doctor is unable to confirm acid reflux as the source of the problem with this test, he may recommend a 24-hour esophageal pH test. The doctor may recommend a barium swallow test if he suspects the symptoms are not acid reflux. (See "Looking at the tests your doctor may run," later in this chapter, for more on the aforementioned tests.)

Infants

Every parent knows it's common for babies to spit up after meals. However, if vomiting is frequent, the infant seems to experience pain or discomfort when feeding, or experiences weight loss, the baby could have acid reflux. Generally, reflux in infants is due to a poorly coordinated gastrointestinal tract. If this is the case, the child will usually outgrow the reflux after her first birthday. In some rare cases, an infant's acid reflux may be due to problems affecting nerves, muscles, or the brain. Be sure to discuss your infant's symptoms with a pediatrician to make sure nothing serious is going on.

Usually, the only acid reflux symptom infants can share is spitting up or vomiting. Although a baby may show signs of discomfort, the stomach acid is usually not strong enough to cause irritation or damage to the esophagus or throat. This means babies usually don't experience heartburn. Reflux often occurs in infants because the LES is not fully developed. They spend most of their time lying flat, which also makes it easier for stomach acid to work its way out of the stomach. Babies' liquid-based diet is another factor that makes them more likely to experience reflux symptoms.

Knowing when to seek medical assistance for your infant's acid reflux is important. Be sure to consult a physician if you notice any of the following symptoms, because they may be a sign of GERD or other more serious medical problems:

- ✔ Weight loss or failure to gain weight
- ✔ Spitting up blood or yellow or green fluids
- ✔ Difficulty breathing or wheezing
- ✔ Blood in the stool or dark stool
- ✔ Frequent vomiting

How Acid Reflux Is Diagnosed

It can sometimes be difficult to figure out if you have acid reflux that's worth worrying about. Just because you have the occasional bout doesn't mean it's anything serious. This is why it's important to keep track of your symptoms and how frequently they occur. A journal can help your doctor figure out if your symptoms are due to acid reflux or something more serious. It can also help the doctor determine the best treatment plan for your symptoms.

Recognizing the symptoms

The three most common symptoms associated with acid reflux and GERD are

- ✔ **Heartburn:** Heartburn is a burning pain or discomfort in the upper abdomen or chest. In rare instances, this burning sensation may reach all the way up to the throat.

✔ **Dyspepsia:** Dyspepsia is stomach discomfort. It's usually associated with excessive burping, nausea after eating, and bloating.

✔ **Regurgitation:** Regurgitation occurs when food, liquid, or bile backs up into your throat. In more extreme cases, this can lead to vomiting.

Acid reflux may also cause a sour or bitter taste in your mouth because of regurgitation. In more serious cases, acid reflux can damage the esophagus and throat, making it difficult to swallow, and can occasionally cause bleeding.

Knowing when to get checked out

If you find yourself experiencing reflux symptoms two or more times a week, it's a good idea to talk with your physician, because you could have GERD. GERD is a chronic digestive disease associated with acid reflux and heartburn that can sometimes lead to serious medical complications such as ulcers, Barrett's esophagus, and even esophageal cancer.

If you're taking over-the-counter medications more than twice a week to deal with reflux, make an appointment to discuss your symptoms with your doctor. It's also a good idea to talk with your doctor if you notice that your symptoms are increasing in frequency or severity. In these instances, you don't need to seek immediate medical attention — just call your doctor and schedule an appointment whenever it's convenient for you.

Call 911 if you experience chest pain, especially if it's accompanied by shortness of breath and jaw or arm pain, because these may be signs of a heart attack.

Looking at the tests your doctor may run

Because acid reflux is so common and generally doesn't result in further medical complications, it's common for physicians to diagnose acid reflux based on symptoms alone. If you experience mild or infrequent reflux symptoms, your doctor probably won't want to do any extra testing. This doesn't mean that she doesn't care about your symptoms or that she isn't thorough. She just sees acid reflux cases all the time, so unless she's afraid it's something more serious, like GERD, your doctor will likely avoid uncomfortable and sometimes expensive testing.

That said, there are several different medical tests and procedures that doctors use to help assess the severity of acid reflux or GERD.

Upper endoscopy

Upper endoscopy is a simple and generally painless procedure that can be helpful in diagnosing acid reflux or GERD. It's a quick outpatient procedure, which means you won't have to stay in the hospital. The procedure usually involves light sedation given into your vein. After you're sedated, a doctor will slide a slender tube (with a tiny embedded camera and light) down your throat and esophagus into the stomach. The camera allows the doctor to examine the esophagus and stomach. He can look for and identify any abnormalities or potential problem areas, and also assess the damage that reflux has done to your esophagus. This is usually the only test your doctor will need to confirm a case of acid reflux or GERD.

In some instances, your doctor may want to perform a biopsy. In this case, the doctor will send a tiny pair of tweezers through the endoscope and remove small pieces of tissue from your esophagus for analysis. The tissue samples will be examined by a pathologist using a microscope. This will help assess the reflux-related damage and rule out any other problems or causes.

Bravo pH probe

A Bravo pH probe is a capsule-based test that allows physicians to collect information over multiple days. This text can help them assess the frequency and duration of acid reflux. This test may be recommended if your doctor wants to confirm that your symptoms are the result of GERD and not something else.

Unlike some of the other pH tests, Bravo pH probes are catheter free. During the upper endoscopy procedure, your doctor will temporarily pin a miniature pH capsule to the lower end of your esophagus. This capsule will then transmit information to a small receiver that's worn on a shoulder strap or waistband.

The nice thing about this type of testing is that it allows you to go about your normal daily activities without much inconvenience. During this procedure, you can take off the receiver to shower or sleep without affecting the results. Being able to do your daily routine can also provide your physician with a more accurate picture of your acid reflux.

Impedance pH probe

An impedance pH probe is another type of probe your doctor may recommend. This test is performed to detect reflux activity over a 24-hour period. The test allows physicians to categorize reflux symptoms as either acidic or nonacidic. This can help your doctor assess what types of treatment would be most effective, especially if your current treatment isn't working well. It can also be used after treatment has begun to determine just how effective your current treatment regimen is at controlling your acid. The procedure begins with an esophageal motility test, which allows your physician to determine the correct placement of the probe. During this part of the procedure, a specially trained nurse will insert a small catheter in the nostril down into the stomach. You'll be asked to take small sips of water as the nurse slowly withdraws the catheter.

After the motility test is completed, the nurse will insert the impedance pH probe through your nose, using a different specially designed catheter. This catheter will come out your nose and be attached to the receiver unit. The probe will stay in place for 24 hours, sending information to a special receiver that you'll carry on a strap over your shoulder. You'll have to return the following day to have the probe removed. The nurse will also ask you fill out a diary to record specific events during that 24-hour period.

Pharyngeal pH probe

Your physician may recommend a pharyngeal pH probe if he suspects that your reflux is causing respiratory or laryngeal problems. Typical laryngeal problems associated with acid reflux and GERD include hoarseness, coughing, excessive throat clearing, and asthma.

During this test, your doctor will insert a catheter in the nostril and down into the esophagus, and place the pH probe in a specific location in your esophagus. The probe has two monitors for pH levels; the first is placed just above the LES and the second monitor is located just below the upper esophageal sphincter. This test can help your doctor determine if the abnormal acid exposure is due to acid reflux or something else. If both probes detect high levels of acid exposure, it's a safe bet that your problems are due to acid reflux. If only the lower probe detects increased acid exposure, it can be a sign that your laryngeal symptoms may be the result of some other problem.

Esophageal motility testing

If you have difficulty swallowing, your doctor may recommend esophageal motility testing, otherwise known as esophageal manometry. This test measures the esophagus function, as well as LES function. During this procedure, the motility nurse will insert a small, flexible catheter through your nostril down into the esophagus and stomach. Over a period of about 20 minutes, she'll slowly withdraw the catheter. The nurse will ask you to swallow frequently throughout the procedure. This enables the medical staff to measure the pressure at different points in your esophagus. The catheter is attached to a device that records these measurements for analysis. Don't worry though — this catheter only remains in your nose for less than a half hour!

This test can help your physician determine whether your difficulties swallowing are due to acid reflux or something else. The procedure can also be helpful in determining the most effective treatment regimen for your acid reflux or GERD.

Chapter 3

Recognizing the Dangers of the Condition

In This Chapter
▷ Identifying the possible complications associated with acid reflux
▷ Assessing and reducing your risks

A wide variety of medical complications can develop as a result of acid reflux. Some of these can be life-threatening, and even those that aren't life-threatening can be life-altering. They can force you to change your daily routines or lead to expensive and sometimes dangerous medical treatments.

Regardless of whether the consequences are severe or simply a nuisance, the first step is to learn the risks and how best to reduce them. The more you understand about your battle with acid reflux and its complications, the more likely you are to control it.

Seeing What Can Happen If Acid Reflux Isn't Treated

Most people will experience heartburn or acid reflux at some point in their lives, so it may not seem like it's a very big deal. You may see it as a minor, occasional inconvenience at worst. Even those who face reflux and heartburn on a regular basis may simply consider it a part of life that they just have to deal with. Reflux usually does not lead to serious or life-threatening complications. But no matter how normal your reflux may seem, treating it is important so that you're more comfortable and so that you reduce the risk of complications.

You don't need to worry if you only have heartburn or reflux symptoms once or twice a year. However, if that were the case, you probably wouldn't be reading this book. If you have reflux more than a couple times a year, mention it to your physician at your next annual checkup. Early awareness and prevention can help ensure that you don't develop any of the more serious long-term complications associated with acid reflux.

Ignoring your symptoms, no matter how small, can lead to a variety of issues. In some severe cases, untreated reflux can lead to cancer and death. Ignoring symptoms can not only make your suffering worse but also lead to financial and personal complications. If your reflux goes untreated long enough, it can cause severe damage to your esophagus, larynx, and even your teeth. Left untreated, your reflux itself can get worse, which may result in the need for corrective surgery. And as anyone who has ever spent even a night in the hospital knows, medical care is extremely expensive.

If you're reading this book, you're proactive, and unlikely to end up in those dire straits. Congrats!

Semi-serious stuff

Yes, acid reflux can rob you of sleep and lead to irritability and difficulty concentrating. Dealing with chronic pain or exhaustion from a lack of rest can be extremely difficult, but none of that is as important as some greater complications.

Over time, exposure to stomach acid (now that's some corrosive stuff) can lead to irritation and inflammation of the esophagus. This irritation and even ulceration in the esophagus is called *esophagitis,* and it can be a precursor to more significant, even life-threatening complications, such as Barrett's esophagus. Even if it doesn't develop into something more serious, esophagitis is serious enough on its own, because it causes discomfort, nausea, vomiting, and difficulty swallowing.

The damage that reflux can do to your throat and larynx can lead to other complications as well. You may have noticed that bad bouts of reflux have left your throat irritated and inflamed. This irritation can cause chronic coughing, choking, hoarseness, and even difficulty speaking. It can also affect your lungs, leading to breathing problems and increasing the severity of existing health conditions like asthma.

Acid reflux can even have an impact on your teeth. Stomach acid is strong enough to damage and destroy tooth enamel. If you suffer from reflux on a regular basis, you may have noticed tooth discoloration or increased sensitivity to hot and cold. In severe cases, reflux can do so much damage to enamel that it results in tooth extractions.

In this section, we cover other semiserious complications of acid reflux.

Reliance on antacids: Not a good thing

You've probably taken antacids at some point in your battle with acid reflux. The effectiveness of antacids varies from person to person. Although antacids may eliminate all discomfort for some people, other people get no relief from antacids. Either way, antacids are the most common way people deal with heartburn and reflux symptoms. In fact, antacids are one of the most widely used and best-selling pharmaceutical drugs in the world.

Antacids are not designed to cure acid reflux or address the root cause of it. They're intended to relieve the discomfort and pain associated with stomach acid by temporarily neutralizing it.

A large variety of antacids are on the market, but all of them work by neutralizing or absorbing stomach acid. This makes the overall symptoms, especially heartburn, less severe. If you have occasional acid reflux, your doctor will likely recommend antacids. Antacids are so common that it's easy to think they're harmless. However, antacids do have some risks associated with long-term use:

- **Antacids may prevent you from addressing the actual cause of your reflux.** Because antacids only treat the symptoms, some more serious conditions may go undiagnosed. And long-term, untreated acid reflux can lead to serious health complications that may even result in death.

- **Most antacids contain either aluminum hydroxide or magnesium hydroxide, to help neutralize and absorb stomach acid, and these compounds can have serious side effects.** There are concerns that large quantities of either compound have been linked to memory loss and early-onset senility. Both of these potentially permanent side effects can have a terrible impact on quality of life.

  The chemicals aluminum hydroxide and magnesium hydroxide have also been linked to:

  - Diarrhea
  - Excessive tiredness
  - Loss of appetite
  - Muscle pain
  - Swelling
  - Weakness

Long-term use of these chemicals may contribute to kidney stones, dementia, and Alzheimer's disease.

✔ **Antacids can play a role in reducing your body's ability to absorb essential vitamins and nutrients.** This happens because stomach acid plays an integral role in the absorption of substances such as vitamin B12, magnesium, and calcium. Because antacids neutralize stomach acid, you absorb less of these essential nutrients. Over the long term, a lack of B12 can damage your central nervous system. This leaves you more likely to develop dementia, neurological damage, or anemia.

✔ **Antacids may make your reflux worse.** In some cases, antacids can actually lead to a phenomenon called *acid rebound,* which happens when your stomach reacts by producing more acid, which in turn magnifies the severity of your reflux symptoms.

Despite all the potential side effects, antacids can be an effective and safe treatment for many people who suffer from acid reflux. Taking antacids for the occasional bout of heartburn is very unlikely to lead to any of these complications.

However, frequent, long-term use or abuse of antacids can have significant health risks. Be sure to discuss antacid use with your doctor, especially if you use antacids for more than two weeks.

Cough

Coughing may not sound like a big deal. We all have a cough from time to time. Yes, it can hurt and make your throat feel raw and dry, but it'll feel better in a few days, right? Unfortunately, this is not the case for many people with acid reflux–related coughs.

First, the discomfort and irritation that results from constant coughing can be more severe. This makes sense because your throat may already be irritated, inflamed, or damaged by stomach acid and enzymes that have splashed up.

Second, many people with reflux-related coughs have what is known as a *chronic cough.* Chronic coughs are persistent. It's something that you'll have to deal with every day, and unfortunately for many people, it won't go away anytime soon, maybe ever. Although some patients have been lucky enough to eliminate a chronic cough with treatment, many others haven't.

Imagine not being able to sleep because your cough keeps waking you up. Imagine not being able to go to the movies or out to a nice restaurant because you're worried that your constant coughing is going to ruin the experience for others. Or imagine what it must feel like to have people stare at you, wondering what illness you have that is making you cough so much, and whether you're contagious. Maybe all this is the case for you, and you don't have to imagine at all.

Not every chronic cough is the result of acid reflux, but between 20 percent and 40 percent of chronic coughs are believed to be related to acid reflux or gastroesophageal reflux disease (GERD). There are two primary reasons why acid reflux causes coughing. The first reason is due to stomach acid itself; if even a small amount of stomach acid reaches the larynx or gets into the lungs, it can trigger a coughing spell. The other reason is due to automatic reflexes, which developed as the digestive track evolved; a little bit of reflux in the esophagus can trigger an automatic reflex that induces coughing.

One significant issue that physicians face is being able to diagnosis chronic cough as a result of acid reflux. Although it's possible to have symptoms like heartburn, many patients with reflux-related chronic coughs do not experience the more common symptoms of reflux. Because a patient may not be experiencing other reflux symptoms, it's quite easy for her doctor to overlook reflux as a potential cause.

There are two primary ways in which your doctor will try to verify that a cough is the result of reflux:

- **pH testing:** This procedure allows physicians to verify that stomach acid is making it into the top portion of the esophagus and can help quantify the severity of the reflux and the association between reflux episodes and cough.

- **Proton pump inhibitor (PPI) therapy:** In this test, you'll be given high doses of PPIs (drugs that reduce gastric acid production) while your cough symptoms are monitored for up to three months. If your cough improves during this time, you'll likely be diagnosed with a reflux-related chronic cough.

Hoarseness

Just like coughing, it's common for people with reflux to experience hoarseness. Hoarseness can be extremely uncomfortable. If you've ever had to clear your throat while you were sick, you can start to understand what chronic hoarseness can feel like. It's that same feeling of not wanting to swallow or cough for fear of the searing pain, only now it's a daily struggle.

And it's not only how you *feel* that'll be affected, but how you *sound.* You may be hoarse without pain at all. You may experience a change of pitch or volume in your voice. In some cases, a voice will get deeper or harsher. Your voice can sound gravelly or scratchy. You may even lose your voice completely as a result of acid reflux's impact on your vocal cords. This is one reason why acid reflux is a huge problem for professional singers. Not only can it change the overall tone and quality of the voice, but the acid can damage the vocal cords.

When acid reflux reaches the larynx or throat, it's known as larynogopharyn-geal reflux (LPR). When vocal-fold swelling is combined with cough (another common symptom associated with LPR), it can lead to vocal-fold lesions. These also damage the voice. In many cases, vocal lesions can only be repaired through surgery.

There is some encouraging information when it comes to hoarseness related to reflux and LPR. First, LPR is less common than acid reflux. It's more dif-ficult for stomach acid to travel all the way up the esophagus to the larynx and throat. In some cases, stomach acid will only reach the larynx and throat when you're lying down. This is why many people who deal with acid reflux–related hoarseness complain that their symptoms are worse in the morning.

The other piece of good news is that, unlike reflux-induced chronic coughing, treatment for hoarseness is generally more effective. The first step is usually to treat the acid reflux. Several studies have shown that medication com-monly taken to treat reflux or GERD eliminates hoarseness after just a few weeks.

If you're experiencing hoarseness, rest your voice as much as possible. This will minimize the damage to your vocal cords and give them time to heal and recover. Also, do your best to avoid irritants such as dust, chemical fumes, tobacco smoke, or alcohol.

Gastroesophageal reflux disease

GERD is a more serious, chronic, or longer-lasting form of acid reflux. Although heartburn and acid reflux are extremely common, with almost everyone experiencing them at least once, GERD is less prevalent.

Approximately 15 million Americans report experiencing GERD symptoms on a daily basis. GERD can be a tremendous nuisance, affecting your quality of life and limiting your daily activates, but it's rarely life-threatening. And in many cases, proper treatment and care can minimize or even eliminate GERD.

GERD is a digestive disorder that affects the lower esophageal sphincter (LES). The LES is a ring of muscles that separates the esophagus and the stomach. When it's functioning properly, it opens to allow food and fluids to pass into the stomach and then closes, preventing any of the stomach contents from flowing back into the esophagus. When it's not functioning properly, the LES allows the stomach contents to escape back into the esophagus, which is known as acid reflux. The severity of GERD is dependent on just how dysfunc-tional a person's LES is, on how much stomach acid is brought up from the stomach, and on how long that acid remains in the esophagus.

A variety of factors contribute to the development of GERD:

- Alcohol use
- Hiatal hernia
- Obesity
- Pregnancy
- Smoking
- Some medications

The symptoms associated with GERD are the same as for acid reflux. In most cases, the only difference is the severity and frequency of the symptoms.

There are several ways that doctors treat GERD. One way is through lifestyle changes. These include losing weight, quitting smoking, cutting out alcohol, and changing the diet. The most common dietary changes involve reducing meal size and avoiding certain trigger foods. In some cases, doctors prescribe medication to treat GERD. In very rare circumstances, GERD treatment requires surgery. Surgery will only be considered an option after all other potential treatments have been ruled out.

You may feel like you can manage your GERD on your own, but it's important to talk with your doctor about your symptoms. Left untreated, long-term GERD can lead to more serious health complications. One of the most common is *esophagitis* (inflammation and ulceration of the esophagus), which can lead to bleeding, or food getting stuck when you're trying to swallow. GERD can also contribute to respiratory problems, including asthma. In the most serious cases, GERD can lead to the development of Barrett's esophagus, a condition that can turn into esophageal cancer (covered later in this chapter).

Sleep disturbance

One of the most common complaints doctors hear from patients with acid reflux is that it messes with their sleep. Whether they toss and turn and can't fall asleep, or wake up with pain in the middle of the night, acid reflux can be a nightmare. In fact, most people complain that their heartburn or other acid-reflux symptoms are worse at night, especially right before bedtime.

This makes sense for several reasons. For starters, most people tend to make dinner their biggest meal of the day. Large meals stretch the stomach too much and put more pressure on the LES, often leading to heartburn. Second, we're all more likely to lean back or lie down after dinner than at other meals. Remove gravity from the mix and it's easier for acid to shoot up into the esophagus. Because most people lie down to sleep, this is a recipe for discomfort.

Having your sleep interrupted occasionally may not seem like a big deal, but it can actually have a tremendous impact on your overall happiness and health. Study after study has shown that sleep deprivation leads to irritability, increased stress, and difficulty concentrating. A few missed nights of sleep can quickly lead to problems at work and in personal relationships, and a lack of sleep can also affect physical health. Studies have shown that failing to get enough sleep (around eight hours a night) can lead to a variety of health risks including obesity, heart disease, diabetes, headaches, depression, and in severe cases, even death.

But don't freak out — there are several steps you can take to minimize the impact reflux has on your sleep patterns:

- **Avoid lying down for at least two hours after you eat.** This will give your stomach more time to digest your meal, and make it less likely that stomach acid will enter your esophagus.

- **Try to make dinner one of the smallest meals of the day.** This will speed stomach emptying and decrease the amount of pressure on your LES. Limit your fat content at that meal, too — fat slows the emptying of the stomach and can lead to increased reflux.

- **Elevate the head of your bed, use a foam bed wedge, or prop a few pillows under your shoulders and down to your hips to incline your body when you go to sleep.**

- **Wear loose-fitting clothes to bed.** This will reduce the pressure on your stomach.

- **Sleep on your left side.** Studies have shown that sleeping on the left side helps with gastric emptying. Many reflux patients have found that this also reduces the frequency and severity of nighttime reflux attacks.

Super-serious stuff

Some of the less serious side-effects (see the previous sections) can have a profound impact on your day-to-day life, but it's the super-serious complications you really need to worry about. Often, they're the result of not treating acid reflux or GERD. Most of these complications are the result of long-term reflux, not the occasional bout.

As we explain in this section, many of the symptoms associated with the more serious complications are the same as or similar to acid reflux. Because of this, determining if your symptoms are the result of reflux or something more serious can be difficult. That's why it's important to be very specific when you're telling your doctor about the types and severity of symptoms you experience. The more accurate and specific the information your doctor has, the more likely she is to be able to identify the problem in time to do something about it.

Your doctor can make you aware of any other health risks associated with acid reflux. If you catch any of the serious complications early enough, that vigilance may save your life.

Aspiration pneumonia

Aspiration pneumonia is an inflammation of the lungs and bronchial tubes. It results from inhaling vomit, food, or liquid. While this can happen to anyone, people with acid reflux are at a heightened risk for developing it. This is because reflux makes it possible for the stomach's contents to make it up the esophagus, through the larynx, between the vocal cords, and into the lungs. Aspiration pneumonia is actually a very common form of pneumonia, accounting for approximately 15 percent of all pneumonia cases. It's more commonly found in men, young children, and the elderly, or those who are weakened by health issues.

A variety of symptoms are associated with aspiration pneumonia. The most common symptoms are

- ✔ Bluish tint of the skin
- ✔ Chest pain
- ✔ Coughing
- ✔ Fatigue
- ✔ Fever
- ✔ Gurgling
- ✔ Shortness of breath
- ✔ Wheezing

Talk with your physician immediately if you notice any of these symptoms. It's important to seek immediate medical attention for this condition. That attention can have a real impact on the effectiveness of the treatment and your likelihood for recovery.

When caught quickly, aspiration pneumonia usually won't lead to further complications. Still, several other factors influence the effectiveness of treatment, including what percentage of your lungs has been affected, the severity of the pneumonia, as well as the type of bacteria that caused the infection.

Treatment usually starts with a round of antibiotics. The specific type of antibiotics that'll be effective depends on the type of bacteria causing the infection, and this can be difficult for doctors to identify. In some cases, depending on the severity of the infection and symptoms, patients may require hospitalization. Doctors continue antibiotic treatment and attempt to alleviate any other symptoms.

Without treatment, the consequences can be devastating. Two common complications are associated with aspiration pneumonia:

- ✔ **Lung abscess:** A lung abscess is a pus-filled cavity in the lungs that causes severe pain and difficulty breathing.
- ✔ **Acute respiratory failure:** Acute respiratory failure occurs when fluid builds in the air sacs in your lungs. When that happens, your lungs can't release oxygen into your blood. In turn, the organs can't get enough oxygen-rich blood.

Be sure to speak with your physician immediately or go to urgent care or the nearest emergency room if you start showing symptoms of aspiration pneumonia.

Stricture

An esophageal *stricture* is a narrowing of the esophagus due to a buildup of scar tissue. Most esophageal strictures are benign (noncancerous), but a stricture can become cancerous. Whether the stricture is cancerous or benign, it should be taken seriously because it can lead to significant health issues. Here, we focus on benign strictures, because they're much more common.

Acid reflux makes you significantly more likely to develop esophageal strictures than the average person. Acid reflux is actually the primary cause of esophageal strictures. Corrosive stomach acid can do terrible damage to the esophagus and the esophageal lining. If you have reflux, especially GERD, your esophagus is exposed to stomach acid on a regular basis, making it easy to see why you're more likely to incur damage. As the damage heals, it becomes scar tissue, which can lead to a narrowing of the esophageal opening around the scarring. It's fairly common for GERD patients to develop strictures — up to 23 percent of GERD patients develop them.

Several symptoms are commonly associated with esophageal strictures. The first, and most common, is *dysphagia*. Dysphagia is characterized by difficulty swallowing, or feeling that food is not making it into your stomach. This is generally accompanied by pain when swallowing, regurgitation, heartburn, and unintended weight loss. Dysphagia can prevent you from getting the proper amount of food or fluid necessary for good nutrition, potentially leading to dehydration and malnutrition. It also increases the risk of choking. Solid or dense foods can easily become lodged in the esophagus above the stricture. The food blocking the esophagus may then contribute to *pulmonary aspiration,* which occurs when food or fluids from the stomach enter the lungs. This can lead to aspiration pneumonia (see the preceding section).

Because the symptoms of stricture are commonly associated with acid reflux and some other common health problems, diagnosis usually requires medical testing. There are generally three ways physicians try to confirm an esophageal stricture:

- ✔ **Barium swallow test:** During this test, you undergo a series of X-rays after drinking a barium solution that coats your esophagus. This allows your physician to get a clear picture of the area.

- ✔ **Upper endoscopy:** In this case, an *endoscope* (a small tube with a camera) is inserted into the esophagus to look for any scarring and narrowing. This procedure allows physicians to take a sample of the damaged area and do a biopsy to determine its underlying cause. The structured area may be dilated during this procedure if necessary.

- ✔ **Esophageal pH monitoring:** For this procedure, a specially trained nurse inserts a slender tube or probe with a pH monitor down your nose to dangle in your esophagus; the tube is left taped to your nose and face for the next 24 hours.

  The pH testing results will tell your doctor lots of important information about your GERD, including whether the refluxing material is acid, bile, or neutral stomach contents; when it occurs (like after eating or when you lie down); and if the reflux episodes are associated with your symptoms. It helps your doctor know if your chest pain, your cough, your throat clearing, or your hoarseness occur at the time of your reflux. In addition, your doctor may need to increase your antacid medications.

When a physician has confirmed your esophageal stricture, treatment will begin. The method of treatment will vary depending on the severity, as well as the underlying cause, of the stricture. The most common treatment is *esophageal dilation.* During this procedure, the physician inserts an endoscope with a small, inflatable balloon into the esophagus. When the balloon is at the stricture, the doctor slowly begins to inflate the balloon, which stretches out and widens the damaged area.

Other techniques use a soft rubber dilator inserted over a guide wire that has been placed down the esophagus and into the stomach by endoscopy. Several dilators, of escalating size, will be used to bring the esophagus up to a size less likely to catch food. Repeated dilations may be required, because strictures may slowly narrow again over time.

Rarely, an esophageal stent may be required if the stricture is very tight, long, or keeps closing down. In this case, the doctor will insert a collapsed stent (think of a wire mesh Chinese finger puzzle) into the narrowed area of your esophagus while doing an upper endoscopy. The doctor will deploy the stent, allowing it to expand. Stents are usually removed after a while, having allowed the scarred area to heal around the diameter of the stent. This will keep the area stretched out, while still allowing food and fluid to pass through. Extremely rarely, surgery may be required to remove the damaged area.

In most cases, your doctor will also recommend dietary and lifestyle changes. Because reflux is one of the primary culprits behind esophageal strictures, preventing or reducing reflux symptoms will be important. This may include some prescription medications taken to prevent or reduce reflux or GERD.

Although treatment is important and can be effective, it may not be permanent. In fact, 30 percent of patients who get esophageal dilation will have to have it done again at least two times. When you develop a stricture, you'll likely spend the rest of your life on medication or having to make permanent changes to your lifestyle and diet.

If you take the time to address and manage your reflux early on, you can significantly reduce your chances of ever developing an esophageal stricture.

Barrett's esophagus

Barrett's esophagus is a serious condition that involves the tissue lining the esophagus. The exact cause of Barrett's has not been discovered, but acid reflux, and especially GERD, puts you at a greater risk of developing it. You're not likely to develop Barrett's if you have infrequent or mild reflux, but severe cases of GERD have been shown to significantly raise the risk. GERD doesn't *cause* Barrett's, but it's a risk indicator for its development.

Barrett's is a relatively common condition — between 5 percent and 10 percent of GERD patients develop it. When you have Barrett's, the normal tissue lining your esophagus changes into tissue resembling the lining of your intestines. The condition tends to be more prevalent in older adults. The average age of diagnosis is 55, but it's not always clear how long someone has had Barrett's before diagnosis. Men are twice as likely to develop Barrett's than women, with Caucasian men having the highest risk of developing the condition.

Why does Barrett's matter? Because esophagus lining is like your skin, and it has no protection from acid reflux material. Intestinal lining, on the other hand, secretes mucous and bicarbonate, which offers some protection from acid. This change from one organ to another is scary — it's like your eye becoming a third ear.

With no specific symptoms associated with Barrett's, the condition can be difficult to discover. In order to diagnose it, you'll have to undergo an upper gastrointestinal (GI) endoscopy and biopsy. During this procedure, a small tube is inserted through your esophagus into the stomach and duodenum. This allows your gastroenterologist to examine the esophageal tissue and look for any anomalies. The gastroenterologist may then perform a biopsy by taking small pieces of tissue from the lower esophageal lining for microscopic analysis by the pathologist. Usually the gastroenterologist can suspect that Barrett's changes are present simply by looking at the lower esophagus, which has a reddish appearance rather than the pearly pink of a normal healthy esophagus. If it appears that you have Barrett's, the gastroenterologist will likely take several biopsy samples from various levels of the esophagus.

After Barrett's is diagnosed, it's important for your doctor to continue to monitor the condition on a regular basis, because it can develop into cancer.

The best course of treatment will be determined by your doctor based on several factors, including your symptoms, as well as your overall health. In some cases, medication will be prescribed. Usually, it will be a PPI commonly used to combat acid reflux or GERD.

Although PPI treatment may be helpful, there's little evidence that it will reduce your risk of Barrett's developing into cancer. If you've got a long length of Barrett's, or your Barrett's has *dysplasia* (a pathology finding meaning that it is becoming bizarre looking under a microscope and is even closer to becoming cancer), or if you have a family history of esophageal cancer, your doctor will suggest one of the following:

- ✔ **Endoscopic ablative therapy:** This procedure involves burning the Barrett's out of the lining of your esophagus, and allowing normal esophagus lining to regrow in that area. There are two types of endoscopic ablative therapies used to treat Barrett's:

  - **Photodynamic therapy (PDT):** During this procedure, you're injected intravenously with a light-activated chemical called Photofrin. A day later, your doctor will use a laser attached to an endoscope to activate the Photofrin in the affected areas of your esophagus. Once activated, the Photofrin will produce a form of oxygen that destroys the surrounding cells.

    In this way, your doctor can cook the esophagus cells using light-activated chemicals. However, a drawback is that your entire body is photosensitized. You'll need to use extensive sun protection after the injection, until the doctor says you're safe. Think vampire.

  - **Radiofrequency ablation (RFA):** This procedure uses radio waves to a similar effect. Again, an endoscope is used, this time with a balloon with a lacy wire around it that delivers heat energy to the infected area, destroying the surrounding cells. The dead tissue is scraped off, and then the RFA is applied again.

✔ **Endoscopic mucosal resection (EMR):** During this procedure, your physician carefully lifts the abnormal esophageal lining and injects a special solution. After a short period, suction is applied to the abnormal area, which is sliced off and removed. EMR is usually used when there is a specific area of your Barrett's that is of concern, and your doctor needs to remove a chunk deeper than can be burned off with the other techniques. EMR may be used along with PDT or RFA.

In all these treatments, doctors hope to eliminate all the affected cells. After those cells are removed, your body can begin replacing them with normal esophageal cells. In some severe cases, especially if the cells have been confirmed as cancerous, your doctor asks a thoracic surgeon to remove the esophagus entirely.

Esophageal cancer

The big C is a terrifying proposition. The odds of developing esophageal cancer are quite slim, but your odds of surviving a battle with it are slim as well. Each year, around 18,000 people will be diagnosed with esophageal cancer, and around 15,000 people will die from it. But just because the survival rate is low, doesn't mean that you can't beat it.

Types of esophageal cancer

Esophageal cancer usually forms initially in the tissue lining your esophagus. It can have several causes, but long-term acid reflux or GERD puts you at a greater risk of developing the disease. There are two main types of esophageal cancer:

✔ Squamous cell carcinoma, which begins in the flat cells lining the esophagus

✔ Adenocarcinoma, which begins in the cells that produce and release mucus and other fluids in the top part of the stomach where it joins to the esophagus

Both types of cancer are serious and have a high mortality rate.

Cancer occurs when damaged or mutated cells begin to reproduce and spread. As the cells spread, they form tumors. Left unchecked, they can continue to spread to other parts of the body. It's important to note that cancer can form anywhere along the esophagus, but it most often develops in the lower portion of the esophagus. Because the lower part of your esophagus is exposed to more stomach acid when you have reflux, it's understandable that this area would be more likely to be severely damaged. The more often it's damaged and has to repair itself, the greater the risk for cancerous mutation.

How esophageal cancer is diagnosed

Aside from people diagnosed with Barrett's esophagus, it's hard to identify other high-risk groups. Reflux and GERD increase your risk, but the odds of developing esophageal cancer as a result are still quite low. Screenings are not done routinely. This is because of the costs associated with the procedures that diagnose esophageal cancer, and because it's not clear which groups are at high risk. In order to diagnosis esophageal cancer, your doctor will likely perform either an endoscopy or a barium X-ray, both of which are described early in this chapter.

Consult with your doctor if you have any indication that you have esophageal cancer. The cancerous tumor growth may block or close part of the esophagus, making it difficult to eat or drink. In some cases, depending on the location of the tumor, it can impair your ability to breathe as well. It can also cause esophageal bleeding. In some cases, it can lead to severe weight loss as it becomes more difficult for you to swallow food or fluid. In other cases, it can erode your esophagus, creating a tunnel to your trachea, called a *tracheo-esophageal fistula,* which can cause coughing fits whenever you swallow.

There are four different stages of cancer. The higher the stage number, the more difficult your cancer will be to treat. This does not mean that you won't survive if you have stage IV cancer, but it does mean that you'll be in for a serious battle. In stage I, the cancer is only in the top layers of cells lining the esophagus. In stage II, the cancer has spread deeper into the esophageal lining and may potentially have spread to the nearby lymph nodes. In stage III, the cancer has spread deep into the esophageal wall, as well as surrounding tissues, possibly including other parts of the body. In stage IV, the cancer has spread to other parts of the body, making it much more difficult to treat.

The sooner you catch the cancer, the better your chances of survival. So, don't miss your annual physical, and be sure to seek medical advice about your acid reflux or GERD symptoms, especially if you notice they change in frequency or severity.

Asthma

Asthma and acid reflux often go hand in hand, although the exact link between the two has been hard for physicians to determine. In fact, approximately 75 percent of people who suffer from asthma also experience frequent heartburn or have been diagnosed with GERD. People who have asthma are more than twice as likely to develop GERD as those who don't.

Study after study has shown a link between asthma and acid reflux, but there has yet to be a study that proves a causal link in either direction. Despite the lack of causal evidence, most doctors attribute the development of asthma to reflux or GERD under certain circumstances. For instance, adult-onset asthma is often attributed to complications related to GERD. Your physician may also suspect GERD to be the culprit if you find your asthma attacks occur more often after a meal. If your asthma doesn't respond to the usual forms of treatment, it could be another sign that it's a result of your reflux.

There are two main theories as to how acid reflux causes or worsens a person's asthma. One is that the stomach acid released by reflux can inflame the airways and lungs. This makes you more susceptible and sensitive to outside effects such as cigarette smoke, pollution, dust, and even cold air. The other theory has to do with the impact stomach acid has on nerves in your airway. It's believed that acid in the esophagus can trigger a nerve reflux, causing airways to constrict and making it difficult to breath.

Some medications used to treat asthma can worsen or even trigger acid reflux. The medication most commonly associated with worsening reflux symptoms is theophylline. Bronchodilators have also been shown to weaken the LES, making it more likely to allow material to reflux. If you're taking one of these medications and find that your reflux symptoms are getting worse, consider asking you doctor about different methods of treatment that won't inflame your reflux.

Surgery

In some cases, even without any of the complications discussed earlier, your reflux may be severe enough that your doctor recommends corrective surgery. The good news is that most people are able to control or minimize their symptoms without ever having to go under the knife. However, if you find that medications, lifestyle changes, or dietary changes have little impact on your reflux, you may want to consider surgery. Unfortunately, those who respond best to medical management also have better surgical results. Surgery could also be an option if you develop esophagitis, a benign stricture, or Barrett's esophagus.

Any type of surgery carries risks. Surgery should be considered only after all other treatment options have been exhausted. Most people who undergo surgery will have an endoscopy first. This allows the doctor to verify the need for surgery and offers a blueprint for the procedure.

The most common surgery performed to alleviate persistent reflux is called *fundoplication*. This procedure can be carried out in open surgery or laparoscopically. During fundoplication, your surgeon makes an incision (for open surgery) or several small incisions (for laparoscopic surgery) and then wraps and sews the top section of the stomach around the lower section of the esophagus. Think of a hot dog (the esophagus) wrapped in a bun (the top portion of the stomach, known as the fundus). This tightens the lower esophagus, making it more difficult for the stomach's contents to shoot upward. In most cases, laparoscopic surgery will be the preferred method, because it's less invasive and usually has a shorter, less painful recovery period.

Tracking Your Symptoms

The fact that your heartburn, cough, and trouble swallowing could be a simple case of reflux or a sign that you have an esophageal stricture indicates how important tracking your symptoms is.

Paying attention to your symptoms doesn't mean rattling off the few things you remember experiencing on your next trip to the doctor. It means keeping track of not only the types of symptoms you experience, but also their frequency and severity. You should pay close attention to any changes to your regular symptoms. If you suddenly find that you're coughing more often than usual, it may be time for a trip to the doctor. But remember, you don't need to panic if new symptoms start to develop or change. Acid reflux and GERD are quite common, and the vast majority of people with these conditions do *not* face life-threatening consequences.

Next time you take a trip to your doctor, do your best to accurately describe your symptoms including their frequency and severity. It may help to write them down or keep a diary. Be sure to mention any new symptoms that have developed or if any of your old symptoms have disappeared. The more information you can provide your doctor with, the more effectively he'll be able to treat your symptoms.

Rating your discomfort

Objectively describing the severity of your symptoms can be difficult. Most people can tell if their symptoms are getting better or worse, but the impact of each symptom can be very subjective. Each person has a different level of pain tolerance — what one person considers a mild annoyance, another will find unbearable. This makes it almost impossible for doctors to assess your symptoms and determine an appropriate treatment without some sort of standardized pain scale.

Pain scales allow doctors to get a good understanding of how bad your pain is and allow them to compare your pain to that of similar patients. The most commonly used pain scale is a numerical scale. In numerical scales, patients rank their pain from 1 to 10, with 10 being the most severe. There are also verbal pain scales, which use descriptive words to paint a picture of your pain. Finally, there are observational pain scales, which are most often used for patients who are unable to communicate. In this situation, an outside observer, usually the physician, makes judgments based on facial expressions, body language, and physiological features, such as blood pressure and heart rate.

A well-defined point scale can be the most objective and effectively provide your physician with an accurate picture of your pain level. In general the numerical pain scale looks something like this:

- ✔ **1–3:** The pain is mild and doesn't interfere with your day-to-day activities.
- ✔ **4–6:** The pain is noticeable enough that it begins to affect your daily routine.
- ✔ **7–10:** The pain is so debilitating that it stops you from doing most activities other than managing the pain.

Whatever pain scale you end up using, it's important to describe your symptoms and pain level as accurately as possible. Don't exaggerate your pain to elicit sympathy or underrate your pain to seem tough. Be sure to describe how the pain affects your life. Even if two people rate their pain at 9, they may require vastly different treatments. The pain may objectively rate at a 9 for both, but one patient may experience it only for a brief time, which would have little to no impact on daily life. That's very different from someone who faces severe pain for hours on end.

Bottom line: The more accurate the information your doctor receives, the more accurate the diagnosis and treatment will be.

Assessing your risk

When looking at how common acid reflux and GERD are, it seems as though risk is all around us. The fact that 44 percent of people in the United States suffer from heartburn at least once a month and that 20 percent suffer from heartburn at least weekly highlights the reality of this point. But with proper treatment, you're much less likely to develop many of the reflux-related complications. Reducing reflux can get you back to your daily routine and help prevent further health complications.

The risk factors for any of the complications discussed earlier in the chapter vary, but one thing is true of all of them: The longer you have reflux, the more likely you are to develop a complication. This is highlighted by the fact that people with Barrett's esophagus see their odds of getting esophageal cancer go up every year by 0.5 percent. The same is true for many of the other complications related to acid reflux and GERD.

Each person is different, but there are a few things you can work on changing to reduce your risk of acid reflux and its complications:

- ✔ **Keep your weight in check.** Carrying around excess weight puts your body under extra stress and increases the likelihood you'll develop reflux.

- ✔ **Watch your eating habits.** This includes the types of foods you eat and drink, as well as the size and number of meals you have daily. Sometimes a small change in your daily routine can be all it takes to significantly reduce your risk for medical complications.

- ✔ **Realize that age matters when it comes to medical risk factors.** The older you get, the higher your risk. But just because you're young, or have a healthy routine, doesn't mean you're immune. Take your acid reflux and GERD seriously — timely treatment can severely reduce your risk for complications.

Chapter 4

Digesting the Gastrointestinal Triggers (Or Not!)

In This Chapter

▶ Understanding the digestive process

▶ Identifying potential trigger foods

▶ Finding medications that can help with acid reflux

Y ou've probably noticed that certain types of food and drink cause your reflux to flare while others don't. It could be a spicy curry dinner, french fries, or an after-dinner drink. One type of food will trigger your reflux, while that same food may have little to no effect on another person. It can all be very confusing. This chapter will help you figure out what your trigger foods are, and how diet choices play into digestion.

Understanding How Diet Helps

Before we dig into the foods that trigger reflux, it's important to have a general understanding of the overall digestive process. And more specifically, where it goes wrong for people who suffer from acid bound north.

The digestion process

Digestion begins as soon as you take your first bite. When you chew, your teeth break down the food into smaller chunks that will be easier for your body to digest. Saliva also plays a critical role; the chemicals in it start to break down carbohydrates. You swallow, and the food travels down your esophagus. The esophagus is ground zero for acid reflux. It's a long muscular tube that extends from your throat to your stomach.

The esophagus uses a series of muscular contractions, known as *peristalsis,* to push food down into the stomach. Right before the food hits your stomach, it encounters the lower esophageal sphincter (LES), which is a group of muscles that act as a valve. The LES allows food to pass into the stomach but blocks the stomach's contents from creeping back into the esophagus. Figure 4-1 is an illustration of the esophagus, LES, and stomach.

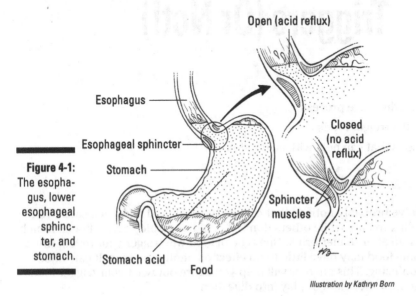

Figure 4-1:
The esophagus, lower esophageal sphincter, and stomach.

Illustration by Kathryn Born

This little valve plays a critical role. If it functions correctly, it prevents stomach acid, enzymes, and food particles from entering the esophagus. In other words, if the LES is doing its job, no reflux.

The next step in the digestive process occurs in the stomach. The stomach is lined by strong muscular walls that expand as food enters. The more you eat, the more the stomach must expand. When the stomach expands, it puts more pressure on the LES. This increased pressure can overcome the LES. You know what that means.

The stomach is also responsible for grinding the food down until it's the correct consistency to pass farther down the digestive tract. The stomach works like a tumbler, pulverizing the food down to sand-sized *chyme.*

From there, the food passes through other organs of the digestive system. Each organ plays its part, further breaking down the food, sucking out the nutrients, and converting the rest into waste.

When digestion goes bad

When the digestive system malfunctions, the results can range from irritating to traumatic. One surprisingly common problem is failing to sufficiently chew food. Just because you can swallow that piece of chicken without chewing, doesn't mean you should. When you don't chew enough, you make it harder on your esophagus and stomach.

If the food is too big and chunky, it may make reflux more painful if you already have it. And if you've developed a narrowing, or stricture, of the esophagus, the chunks may get caught on their journey to the stomach. Failing to fully chew your food also means your stomach has to work harder and take longer to break food down. This digestive distress can make it easier for reflux to rear its ugly head.

The most common complaint associated with acid reflux is heartburn. Heartburn is the result of stomach enzymes and acid getting into the esophagus, causing a burning sensation in the chest. The pain can be so severe that some people mistake it for a heart attack, especially those who aren't used to heartburn. More consequences: excessive burping and a sour or bitter taste in the mouth.

The stomach produces hydrochloric acid and other powerful enzymes to break down the stomach's contents. To prevent the acid from eating away at your stomach lining, your stomach is coated in a thick layer of mucus. If your body produces too much stomach acid, you can face problems like acid reflux or ulcers, but if it produces too little acid you can experience a buildup of small intestinal bacteria, have a greater susceptibility for food poisoning, or have difficulty in absorbing calcium, iron, magnesium, or vitamin B12.

Food Reactions: Listening to Your Body

Even foods that are generally considered healthy, like citrus, garlic, or tomatoes, can turn into your worst enemy if you suffer from acid reflux.

Consider a patient, who prided herself on being very health conscious, and was on a strict diet. You can imagine her surprise when she started to experience severe bouts of heartburn. She was concerned because it wasn't one specific style of food that was triggering her heartburn symptoms. Her doctor dug a little deeper into the patient's diet and realized that her symptoms flared whenever she ate something with raw onions in it.

Your reflux may not be triggered by your favorite type of food, but actually by a single ingredient in the food. This could be the difference between never having another meal in your favorite Chinese restaurant or simply having to switch to beef with broccoli instead of the Kung Pao chicken.

To get to the bottom of this, keep a food journal for at least a week. Be sure to write what type of cuisine you were eating and list as many of the ingredients as possible. Keep track of how you felt after your meal as well. Did your reflux kick in, get worse, or diminish?

Identifying Trigger Foods

The first step in reducing and potentially curing your acid reflux and its symptoms is to identify the foods that trigger it. (More on those foods later in this section). After you've identified the cause of your suffering, the next step is to cut that food out of your life, or at least cut down on it. This can be as simple as avoiding one or two troublesome ingredients. Or maybe the ingredient will be okay with lunch, but not dinner or a midnight snack.

What follows is a list of the most common food types that have been shown to cause or intensify acid reflux.

The corrosive C's

The first group of foods you need to be aware of are the corrosive C's. These foods and drinks are known to trigger reflux symptoms, including heartburn and burping:

- Caffeine
- Chocolate
- Citrus
- Canned foods

You don't necessarily have to avoid all these foods, but you should be aware of the impact they can have on your reflux, and at least consider cutting down on them.

Caffeine

Fifty-four percent of adults in the United States drink at least one cup of coffee a day. Unfortunately, for people with acid reflux, coffee — and more specifically, the caffeine found in coffee — can inflame symptoms.

And it's not just coffee that we get our caffeine from; many sodas and energy drinks are also loaded with caffeine. Tea and even chocolate have caffeine as well.

Caffeinated soda is even worse than coffee. On top of the impact its caffeine has on reflux, you also have to worry about the carbonation. The bubbles from carbonated soda expand inside your stomach, increasing the pressure. This increased pressure can push stomach acid up and out of the stomach, damage your esophagus, and trigger heartburn. Plus, most sodas contain a high level of carbonic acid, which can further irritate your already sensitive esophageal lining.

Caffeine and acid reflux

There are three main ways that caffeine affects reflux:

- ✔ **Caffeine can weaken the LES.** Strength is a critical component for the LES to function properly, and any change, no matter how minor, can cause the LES to malfunction.

    The decreased strength causes the LES to relax. This makes it easier for stomach acid or food particles to sneak back into the esophagus and trigger that terrible burning sensation.

- ✔ **Caffeine causes the stomach to generate more gastric acid.** This is a very strong acid that can do some significant internal damage. The stomach is protected by a thick layer of mucus that prevents acid from damaging or eating through the stomach wall. The esophagus, however, does not have this same protection. So, when gastric acid escapes the stomach, it can wreak havoc on that defenseless esophagus.

- ✔ **Caffeine affects a substance called gamma-amino butyric acid (GABA).** GABA is an important substance produced in the gastrointestinal tract. It plays a crucial role in helping relax the gastrointestinal tract. Caffeine makes GABA less effective, which hampers its ability to act as a relaxing agent in the gastrointestinal tract. GABA also plays a role in helping your body deal with stress. Because stress has been shown to trigger reflux, reducing your ability to deal with stress ups the odds that you'll get acid reflux.

Jitterbug: Living with less caffeine

Caffeine is actually a drug. And just like some drugs, it may be addictive. Quitting or even simply cutting back on caffeine intake can lead to withdrawal symptoms. The severity of these symptoms is often tied to how dependent your body has become on caffeine. Reducing your caffeine intake can lead to a wide variety of physical symptoms, including the following:

- ✔ Anxiety and nervousness
- ✔ Constipation
- ✔ Fatigue
- ✔ Headaches
- ✔ Insomnia
- ✔ Irritability
- ✔ Muscle pains and stiffness
- ✔ Physical shaking

Will reducing caffeine reduce your reflux? The jury is out. Frustratingly, there are many conflicting opinions. If you're convinced that caffeine is contributing negatively to your life, consider cutting down on it or cutting it out all together. Because of the potential physical symptoms, it's important to set up a plan for quitting caffeine. If you only have the occasional cup of coffee or soda, you may be able to quit without symptoms. If you're a caffeine fiend, wean yourself off the stimulant instead of going cold turkey.

Try introducing green tea into your routine instead of coffee or soda. Green tea has a very small amount of caffeine, which will help you cut your intake and reduce the intensity of withdrawal.

Chocolate

Sadly, for those who suffer from acid reflux, chocolate can be one of those nuisance trigger foods. For many people, a life without chocolate is a life not worth living. Well, the good news is that you don't have to stop eating chocolate to reduce reflux. Instead, try cutting back. Even if you have gastroesophageal reflux disease (GERD), if you don't notice reflux symptoms after you eat chocolate, then you don't have much to worry about. Now, if it's a problem for you, why is it a problem?

Chocolate and acid reflux

Just like coffee and soda, chocolate contains caffeine. As we explain earlier in this chapter, caffeine can trigger acid reflux. There is much less caffeine in chocolate than in coffee or colas, but chocolate does contain a stimulate called theobromine, which is also known to trigger reflux.

And it's not just the stimulants in chocolate that can cause you trouble. One of chocolate's primary ingredients is cocoa, which has a proven link to heartburn and other reflux symptoms. Research has also found that eating chocolate causes serotonin to be released into the small intestine. Serotonin is a chemical that has been linked to relaxation. Although relaxation is a good thing in general, unfortunately it's not when it comes to acid reflux. The increased serotonin relaxes the LES, which makes it easier for enzymes and acid to escape.

Chocolate is also very high in fat. Research has indicated that eating high-fat foods can lead to GERD. Just like serotonin, high-fat foods make us feel good, but they also cause the LES to relax. And we know what that means: Here comes heartburn. High-fat foods also slow the emptying of the stomach. This can mean acid and food particles stay in your stomach longer, increasing the chances that your reflux kicks in.

Better chocolate choices

Switching to dark chocolate instead of milk chocolate is a smart move, in more ways than one. Because dark chocolate doesn't have as much fat as milk chocolate, it won't slow your stomach emptying as much. The lower fat content also makes it less likely to weaken your LES. Plus, dark chocolate has some added health benefits. It's a great source of antioxidants, which can reduce your risk for heart disease and other illnesses.

The best way to get your chocolate fix without the risk of heartburn or other reflux symptoms is to switch to white chocolate. White chocolate is the only type of chocolate that doesn't contain cocoa. Because cocoa is one of the primary reasons chocolate has been linked to increased incidents of reflux-related symptoms, cutting back on your cocoa intake can help. True, white chocolate isn't really chocolate (there's no cocoa), and it's still high in fat, but again, the lack of caffeine may help.

If you're open-minded about how you get your sugar fix, fruit is always a great option. Not only is it sweet, but it's also a great source of vitamins and nutrients. Even switching to lower-fat candies like gummy bears, licorice, or jellybeans can help. Because they're lower in fat, they're easier to digest, which makes them less likely to trigger your reflux symptoms. But don't go crazy on them — candy is not healthy.

For many people, the best way to eat chocolate is in cake form. Instead of chocolate cake, try switching to angel food cake. You get your cake (and get to eat it, too) but without the cocoa and extra fat. And if angel food cake isn't sweet enough to quench that sugar craving, top it off with some fresh fruit.

Citrus

Yes, a no-brainer: Citrus fruits have a lot of citric acid. And because we know that acid is the primary culprit behind all the pain and suffering we experience as a result of reflux, that can make citrus a no-no. However, citrus has many health benefits. Its high water content makes it a great low-calorie snack. Plus, it's a fantastic source of vitamin C and other nutrients.

If you've been suffering from reflux for quite some time, you've likely had some bad encounters with citrus. The damage reflux does to the esophagus can make a simple glass of orange juice or a sliver of grapefruit a searing source of pain.

Citrus and acid reflux

Oranges and grapefruits are the two most common forms of citrus that cause reflux-related heartburn. It doesn't matter whether it's the fruit itself or its juice — even a little citrus mixed into a smoothie can be enough to cause acid reflux.

As we mention earlier, citrus contains a high level of citric acid. The stomach is lined with mucus, which helps protect the stomach lining from the harmful effects of acid, but the esophagus isn't so lucky. Even people who don't have reflux have experienced a little discomfort if they ever drank a large quantity of orange juice in one sitting. For those people, the occasional bout isn't a big deal. For people with GERD, however, citrus juice can magnify the intensity of reflux. If your throat and esophagus have already been affected over time, even a weak acid like citric acid can do some real damage.

Eating or drinking citrus on an empty stomach increases the odds that you'll suffer heartburn.

Making lemons into lemonade: Solutions

One of the best ways to minimize the damage of citrus on your acid reflux is to simply avoid citrus all together. Switch over to fruits that have a lower acidic content, such as apples, bananas, and watermelon. These gentle fruits can mean less reflux and heartburn, according to some nutritionists.

If you just can't live without citrus, there are some steps you can take to mitigate the harm. First, try not to eat or drink citrus on an empty stomach. When there is nothing else in the stomach, adding acidic foods or drinks means more acid in the stomach and nothing to absorb it. The more acid in the stomach, the greater the chance that some of it will escape into the esophagus and then, yuck, reflux.

You may still be able to enjoy your favorite types of citrus juices by diluting your juice with water, or by drinking water when you eat a piece of acidic fruit. You can also try mixing your citrus in with some plain yogurt, which will help buffer the acidity in the citrus and help soothe your stomach.

Canned foods

Most people who suffer from reflux have probably learned to stay away from many of the foods we mention earlier, but finding out that canned foods can have an impact on your reflux may be a shock.

Yes, fresh fruits and vegetables taste better and have a higher nutritional content. But getting everything fresh, especially if you purchase organic, is more expensive than picking up something canned. It's not just the cost of fresh produce that can make people turn to canned food; it's also about convenience. You may not have time to stop by the farmer's market every week to procure fresh produce. And even if you do, nothing is more annoying than picking up some delicious fresh fruit only to have it go rotten two days after you get home.

Whether it's the money or the convenience that drives you toward canned foods, you may rethink your position when you realize that it could very well be those cans that are causing your suffering.

Meddlesome metal and acid reflux

The main problem when it comes to canned foods, especially fruits, is that they tend to be more acidic than their fresh counterparts. There is a good reason for this. See, manufacturers add acidity to canned goods because it prolongs the shelf life of products. Additionally, acid helps kill bacteria inside the cans.

You'll want to look out for canned products that say "vitamin C enhanced" or "vitamin C enriched," because this is generally a good indicator that the product is more acidic. Also, check the ingredients for any kinds of acid. Whether it's citric acid or ascorbic acid, any form of acid can impact reflux.

It's not just canned fruits and vegetables that have high levels of acid. Canned drinks, including canned sparkling water, are more acidic. In some cases, there is actually more acid in a canned drink than inside the stomach. The extra exposure to highly acidic foods and beverages can lead to severe throat, larynx, and esophagus damage. This long-term exposure has been linked to serious medical problems beyond reflux. In fact, it has been shown that long-term acid exposure can even lead to cancer.

Scrap metal: Alternatives

The best alternative to avoid the acidity found in most canned foods is to switch to fresh food. Fresh fruits and vegetables taste better anyway, and they're better for you. Frozen fruits and vegetables can also be good alternatives.

There are plenty of ways to help you keep your food fresh longer:

- ✔ **Don't store fruits and vegetables together.** Fruits, which give off high levels of a ripening agent called ethylene, will cause your vegetables to spoil faster.
- ✔ **Punch holes in the bags you store your vegetables in to allow for good air flow.**
- ✔ **Don't pack your vegetables too close together in the fridge.** The closer they are together, the faster they rot.

Fruits can also be preserved in several different ways, such as drying. This maintains many of the nutritional qualities of the original, and dehydrating the foods means they'll have a longer shelf life. Also make yourself aware of which types of fruits need to be refrigerated and which types don't. Berries, citrus fruits, grapes, and peppers all decompose rapidly, so they should be stored in the fridge. However, apples, avocados, mangos, melons, pears, and tomatoes can all be left on the countertop until fully ripened.

Other culprits

Plenty of other foods and ingredients have been linked to acid reflux. Many of these have been shown to inflame reflux. For the most part, consuming the following foods occasionally is not going to lead to a GERD diagnosis. It's only through long-term use and through large servings of them that you'll have problems. That doesn't mean you can't ever try them again, but you should be aware of how they impact your reflux. Then you can decide whether they're worth the risk.

Alcohol

Alcohol is a big troublemaker for those with GERD. A fun night out with friends can quickly backfire in more ways than one. Not only can alcohol trigger reflux, but it can also damage an already sensitive esophagus.

Alcohol doesn't have a high level of acidity. So if it's not the acidity affecting your reflux, what is? It turns out that alcohol, in any form, can make it more difficult for your body to clear acid out of the esophagus. This is especially true when you lie down. Most people with GERD have likely realized that reclining after a meal is a quick way to trigger heartburn, but they may not think twice about it after a few drinks.

Some people drink alcohol during the day, but the majority have their drinks at night. The practice is so common that we even have a term for it: the *nightcap*. Because alcohol can make you tired, it may seem natural to have a drink or two after a meal and then go to bed. But if you have reflux, a nightcap can turn into a nightmare.

Research has shown that any type of alcohol — beer, wine, or liquor — can lead to a night of tossing and turning. The heightened risk of reflux symptoms lasts longer than with food consumption. It's not just a matter of staying upright and awake for two hours like after a regular meal. Research has shown that consuming even a small amount of alcohol three hours before bedtime can still result in a night of heartburn.

How liquor is typically consumed can also increase the chances of a reflux flare-up. Many people, especially when they're at a bar or restaurant, don't drink straight liquor. Instead they'll opt for a cocktail that combines alcohol with some other ingredients, such as juice or soda. And citrus and soda, of course, are reflux no-no's.

Any type of alcohol can cause reflux, but most research indicates that wine and liquor are the most troublesome. That's not to say that having a few beers means you're in the clear. There is evidence that beer consumption still makes you significantly more likely to experience reflux than if you were just drinking water.

Meat

Meat is the primary source of protein in most people's diets. Although you can easily get protein from other sources — primarily beans, nuts, tempeh, and soy — many people shudder at the thought of eating less meat.

Part of why meat is troublesome for people with reflux is that it's hard to grind down to chyme. Because meat is so difficult to digest, it stays in the stomach longer than many other foods. This means the stomach will be expanded for a longer period of time, putting pressure on the LES for a longer period of time. The longer the LES is stressed, the more likely it is that some of the stomach contents will slip up to the esophagus.

Meats with a lot of fat are the worst. High-fat foods sit in your stomach for longer periods of time, stretching the stomach and increasing the pressure put on the LES. This is one of the reasons doctors recommend eating lean proteins such as: beans, fish (cod, flounder, grouper, haddock, halibut, herring, mackerel, mahi-mahi, orange roughy, swordfish, tilapia, trout, tuna, wild catfish), shellfish (crab, lobster, scallops, shrimp), game meat (buffalo, deer, elk), and poultry (chicken, turkey).

Red meat often has a higher fat content and, therefore, is slower to exit the stomach. Cutting out red meat completely may be ideal, but if you can't live without the occasional steak or burger, try to limit your intake of red meat to one red-meat meal every two weeks. When you do get a steak or burger, make the smart choice and go for the leaner cuts, and don't have a big portion.

If you have severe acid reflux, consider cutting back your meat intake in general, to eating meat only two or three times a week. To make up for the lost protein, start incorporating beans, soy, and nuts. Be aware of the serving size for nuts though, because they're high in fat. Limiting to a handful or two is best, or read the label. You'll likely be surprised at the scant number of nuts you should eat per serving.

Fried foods

As delicious as fried foods may be, they're a recipe for disaster when it comes to health. Fried foods are a culprit in many medical issues in the United States. They're linked to obesity and heart disease and, of course, acid reflux.

The worst offender cited in study after study is french fries, followed closely by fried chicken strips. But it isn't just fries and chicken strips that cause reflux and heartburn. Any fried food, including healthy green vegetables battered and fried, can contribute to the problem.

There are several reasons fried foods, especially deep-fried foods, are linked with heartburn and reflux. The first is the extraordinarily high fat content found in fried foods. Foods with a lot of fat stay in the stomach much longer than other types of food, which is a recipe for heartburn and reflux.

And it's not just the fat content found in fried foods that can lead to reflux. Fried foods, just like several of the other foods discussed in this chapter, weaken the LES. Researchers have yet to identify the specific reason that fried foods have this effect, but the link is well documented. Eating fried foods often and in large quantities may set you up for a GERD diagnosis.

Scary spice

A bland meal, blah. One of the main reasons people stray from their diets is due to a lack of flavor. Eating the same bland meals, day after day, can be almost as bad as having to deal with acid reflux. But be careful because many of the spices used to increase flavor can trigger reflux and heartburn.

There are so many different spices and varieties of seasonings that it can be difficult to figure out which ones are the problem. Because people don't consume spices by themselves, figuring out just what's causing reflux is even more challenging. There are however, some general guidelines to follow.

In general, fresh herbs and spices are less likely to trigger reflux than their dried counterparts. This is due to the high levels of preservatives contained in premade spice mixes. Preservatives make the spice and seasoning last longer and also make them harder to digest.

Food doesn't have to be bland, but you should still avoid a heavy hand with the seasoning. Often the stronger the spice, the more likely it is to impact reflux. The spices and seasonings most associated with acid reflux are

- ✔ Cayenne pepper
- ✔ Cloves
- ✔ Chili powder
- ✔ Curry
- ✔ Mustard
- ✔ Nutmeg
- ✔ Pepper (black, cayenne, red, and white)

Herbs such as basil, cilantro, dill, oregano, rosemary, thyme, and even ginger can all add a host of flavor to your food without causing reflux.

Just like many of the other problem foods, the impact that one particular spice or seasoning has on you may not be the same for someone else. That's why it's crucial to pay attention to what kind of spices and seasonings are in your meals. This is fairly easy when you're preparing meals at home, but it can be a challenge when dining out. Don't be afraid to ask your server what spices and seasonings are used to prepare your meal. It's better to feel like a slight nuisance than to go home and lose a good night's sleep to pain because you didn't want to *be* a pain.

Despite all the anecdotal evidence that spicy food triggers reflux, the science isn't certain. Many studies have concluded that spicy food in itself doesn't make you any more likely to suffer from acid reflux or heartburn. It does, however, make you more likely to feel reflux's effects. As with other foods in this book, you'll have to figure out through trial and error what affects your reflux symptoms. Start a diary of foods and symptoms to keep track.

Mint

Mint is found in all types of cuisine. It can also be found in cocktails, such as mojitos. Mint is often used to give a light and refreshing boost to a meal or drink. And there isn't just one type of mint; there are approximately 700 varieties!

Sadly, mint may freshen your breath, but it can also inflame reflux.

Like many of the other troublesome foods, mint can cause your LES to relax. You know what that means: A relaxed LES makes it is easier for stomach acid to sneak by. So, if you're looking for an after-dinner palate cleanser, avoid the mints.

Try switching to licorice, which can be taken in several forms, including chewable tablets. Licorice can actually reduce your risk for heartburn because it contains anise, a spice that aids digestion. Gum can also be a good way to reduce the likelihood of a reflux flare, provided you stay away from the mint flavors. Gum helps because it increases saliva production and causes you to swallow more often. This helps push acid in the esophagus back down into the stomach. And fruit-flavored gum can still freshen your breath after a big meal, without triggering reflux.

Raw garlic

Garlic is another ingredient that's very common in a wide variety of cuisines, and it has several health benefits. It's helpful for reducing the risk for heart disease; plus, it helps you keep those pesky vampires away.

Garlic has an interesting relationship with acid reflux. Some studies have shown that eating cooked garlic can actually reduce reflux symptoms. Whether garlic is helpful or harmful to your reflux depends on how you consume it. Avoid raw garlic, and garlic in chunks.

To be extra safe, some nutritionists suggest that you avoid raw garlic and opt for cooked instead, or simmer food with garlic and then strain it out.

Raw onion

Research has found that raw onion affects only those people who suffer from *chronic* acid reflux. If you rarely experience heartburn or other reflux symptoms, eating raw onions is unlikely to cause you any problems. But if you have GERD, raw onions have been shown to significantly increase the chances you'll suffer from heartburn.

There is some evidence that cooking onions can make them easier to digest. Unfortunately, there have not been enough studies or research to prove this. So, feel free to try foods that have cooked onions in them, but pay attention to how your reflux reacts. If you notice your symptoms flare up afterward, it's a good indicator that you may just want to stay away from onions all together.

Tomatoes

For most people, tomatoes are a good thing. Not only are they nutritional, but they don't contain nearly as much sugar as many other fruits. And just like many of the other troublesome foods we discuss in this section, they're a common ingredient in many cuisines. But because tomatoes are rarely the main component of a meal, many GERD sufferers don't realize tomatoes are a problem.

Tomatoes can be a serious esophageal irritant. Their high levels of acidity can inflame the esophageal lining, leading to reflux. It's not just the high acidity level that's a problem; eating a tomato stimulates the production of extra digestive acids in the stomach. This means you're coping not only with the high acidity of the fruit, but also with the higher acidity level in your stomach. For an already susceptible LES, this can spell trouble.

It doesn't matter what form the tomatoes come in either. Whether they're whole or ground into a paste for a sauce, they can be a nuisance for your reflux.

Cranberry

Cranberries have several health benefits. In fact, cranberries are often used to help prevent and treat urinary tract infections. Not only can they help with many urological issues, but they can kill germs, speed skin healing, reduce fevers, reduce chronic fatigue, and even aid in the treatment of type 2 diabetes.

But for people who have acid reflux, cranberries can spell trouble. Whether consumed whole or in juice form, cranberries can cause acid reflux and heartburn. This is because cranberries contain large quantities of salicylic acid (and acid is the primary culprit behind heartburn).

If you love cranberries and can't imagine Thanksgiving without them, or you use them for the treatment of medical issues, you don't have to cut cranberries out of your diet completely. Here again, moderation is the key. Consumption of small quantities of cranberries is unlikely to cause severe cases of heartburn or have a significant impact on your reflux. If you simply can't live without your cranberry juice, try diluting it with water. And as for Thanksgiving, just take a smaller portion of that cranberry sauce.

Keep it simple

In general, the more complicated a meal is, the harder it may be for your body to digest, according to some registered dietitians. This means your body will have to work harder to break everything down. As part of working harder, it may have to produce more stomach acid, a primary mechanism behind acid reflux.

When a meal is more complex and difficult to break down, it will take longer for your stomach to grind down to small particles. The longer food is in your stomach, the longer your LES is under pressure. If you put even a healthy LES under enough strain for enough time, it will inevitably begin to weaken. This, in turn, allows all that extra stomach acid a chance to escape.

Next time you're planning a meal and you think to yourself, "Wow, there are a lot of ingredients and steps," ask, "If it's this hard to put together in the first place, how hard is it going to for my body to break all this down?" Instead, try to eat meals with just a few simple ingredients and save the complex meals for special occasions. This will make it much easier for your body to digest and reduce your risk for acid reflux.

Factoring in the Meds

Believe it or not, the medications you take also can have an impact on your acid reflux. Fortunately, drugs undergo significant testing for side effects before they go on the market, and the findings are fairly easy to obtain. So yes, you may have to figure it out through trial and error, but the information on which medications may trigger your reflux is available — you'll find it on that piece of paper your pharmacist gives you with your prescription.

Be diligent about monitoring the potential side effects of your medications. Don't rely on your doctor to warn you. Be sure to read the warning labels on any drugs you take, even if you take them only occasionally.

If you find that the medication you're taking lists acid reflux as a possible side effect, don't hesitate to bring it up to your physician or pharmacist. Even if reflux isn't listed as a side effect, let them know if you notice an increase in your reflux symptoms. These medical professionals may be able to offer you an alternative medication that won't impact your reflux.

In this section, we fill you in on some categories of medication that can affect reflux. This list isn't exhaustive, so be sure to continue reading the warnings that come with every medication you take.

Always be sure to discuss your medications with your pharmacist — especially if it's the first time you've taken a particular medication. Ask for a consultation, and don't worry, your pharmacist will probably be happy to discuss your medications with you. Be sure to tell her what other medications you're taking. Don't just bring up your prescription meds — be sure to mention any over-the-counter drugs, vitamins, herbals, or supplements you use as well. And, of course, tell her if you have acid reflux or GERD or experience occasional bouts of heartburn.

Antidepressants

The link between antidepressant medications and acid reflux is somewhat complicated. Some doctors have tried prescribing low levels of antidepressant medication in an attempt to reduce the severity of reflux symptoms. This may help reduce incidents of acid reflux symptoms, but other research has indicated that antidepressants may spur cases of acid reflux.

Research has shown that patients who are long-term users of tricyclic antidepressants are 71 percent more likely to develop GERD than those who are not on the medication. This is because long-term use of tricyclic antidepressants has been shown to relax the LES, a key factor in the development of acid reflux. Although these meds aren't as commonly prescribed as selective serotonin reuptake inhibitors (SSRIs), some physicians still use them for specific cases.

Studies on the more commonly prescribed SSRIs have shown little to no increased risk for GERD. Be sure to check with your doctor about what type of antidepressant medication you're on. If it's a tricyclic antidepressant and you have GERD or you notice an increase in acid reflux symptoms, ask your doctor whether switching to an SSRI is possible.

Anti-anxiety pills

Some anti-anxiety medications have been linked to acid reflux. Certain types can irritate your esophageal lining, leading to more cases of heartburn and increasing the severity of reflux symptoms for those already diagnosed with GERD.

When your esophageal lining is irritated or inflamed, it can magnify the intensity of your reflux symptoms. An already inflamed esophagus will sting more when exposed to the additional irritation caused by acid reflux. It can also put patients with GERD at greater risk for developing more serious esophageal health complications.

Continuous inflammation of the esophagus can cause a buildup of scar tissue. This can make swallowing more difficult and lead to a narrowing of the esophageal opening. This scar tissue is even more sensitive to acid exposure, which means your continued bouts of GERD will become more painful.

As with antidepressants, tricyclic medications are the primary culprit. These types of drugs work by altering the specific neurotransmitters in the brain, helping to reduce or prevent anxiety and panic attacks. The problem is that the stomach has these same neurotransmitters. When these neurotransmitters in the stomach are blocked, that blockage can hinder digestion. It can also cause the LES to relax and become less effective. This combination heightens the chances of developing GERD or experiencing the occasional bout of reflux.

Be sure to check with your doctor about what type of anti-anxiety medication you're taking. If it's a tricyclic and you have GERD or you notice an increase in reflux symptoms, ask whether switching to a different type of medication is possible.

Calcium channel blockers

Calcium channel blockers are a type of medication prescribed to help lower blood pressure. They're used to slow the movement of calcium into the cells of the heart and blood vessel walls, making it easier for the heart to pump while widening the blood vessels. As helpful as these medications can be for blood pressure, they can cause problems for GERD.

Calcium channel blockers can relax the LES. Short-term use of calcium channel blockers is unlikely to cause a problem, but long-term use can. When the LES is continually weakened over a long period of time, it becomes more difficult for muscles to contract after food passes into the stomach.

Many calcium channel blockers can also impact digestion by slowing down stomach emptying. This means more food in the stomach for longer periods of time, which is no good for preventing reflux.

Here are the most commonly prescribed calcium channel blockers that have been liked to acid reflux (the brand names are in parentheses):

- ✔ Amlodipine (Norvasc)
- ✔ Diltiazem (Cardizem, Dilacor, Tiazac)
- ✔ Felodipine (Plendil)
- ✔ Nifedipine (Procardia, Adalat)
- ✔ Nisoldipine (Sular)
- ✔ Verapamil (Verelan, Calan)

Other popular medications

Here are some other types of drugs that have been shown to exacerbate acid reflux:

- ✔ **Bronchodilators:** These are commonly used to treat asthma. Patients taking the inhaled form of bronchodilators had an increased risk of developing GERD.
- ✔ **Hormone replacement therapy drugs:** In one study, women taking estrogen, selective estrogen-receptor modulators, or over-the-counter hormone treatments were 46 percent more likely to develop GERD than women who were not on hormone drugs.

Some other drugs can cause irritation or inflammation in the esophagus, making it more difficult to swallow and making bouts of reflux more painful. Many antibiotics fall into this category. If they're not taken with enough water, there have even been cases where pills lodged in the esophagus, causing chemical burns.

But antibiotics are less worrisome than drugs that you take over long periods of time, such as non-steroidal anti-inflammatories (NSAIDs) or bisphosphonates for osteoporosis. The long-term use of these drugs increases the likelihood of potential side effects that can affect or even cause GERD.

Over-the-counter drugs

It's not just prescription drugs that are linked to acid reflux. Even some common over-the-counter pain relievers have been linked to increased incidents of acid reflux. Some of the most common over-the-counter drugs and supplements that have been linked to GERD include

- Aspirin (Bayer, Bufferin, Excedrin)
- Ibuprofen (Advil, Motrin)
- Iron
- Naproxen (Aleve)
- Potassium
- Vitamin C

Chapter 5

Finding Relief in the Medicine Cabinet and Beyond

- -

- -

*A*cid reflux symptoms vary dramatically from person to person. However, there's one thing that all acid reflux sufferers have in common: They all want relief. Left untreated, even mild cases of acid reflux can do significant, long-term damage to your health and overall quality of life. If your reflux only flares up once a month, that doesn't mean that it's not damaging your esophagus or other parts of your body. And the sooner you choose to act, the better your chances of preventing long-term, potentially life-threatening conditions from developing.

Be prudent about your treatments, and consult your physician. Whether it's an over-the-counter medication, an herbal, or a prescription, keeping your doctor involved in your treatment is essential. Not only can he monitor for any long-term complications, but he can also help ensure that you're treating your reflux in the most efficient, effective way possible.

For many patients, over-the-counter medications will be the starting point in their battle with heartburn and acid reflux. Lifestyle changes are often the most effective method for healing and prevention, but anyone who has suffered a severe bout of reflux can attest to the relief provided by some medications. When you have an intense case of heartburn, a soothing antacid can go a long way toward making life tolerable.

With most medications, including those sold over-the-counter, there are risks associated with long-term use. It's also important to note that most of the treatments for reflux target symptom reduction instead of addressing the cause of the problem. In some cases, the reduction of symptoms may prevent people from seeking medical care or making essential lifestyle changes that could eliminate reflux from their lives.

Keep in mind that even if a particular medication or treatment seems to be working, that doesn't mean that it's the best or most effective treatment. Consult your doctor about any medications you're taking, including over-the-counter meds.

Neutralizing Acid

Antacids are far and away the most commonly used medication to treat heartburn and acid reflux. And it's not only due to their widespread availability; it's also because they're very good at treating heartburn, the most annoying symptom of acid reflux. With about half of adults in the United States reporting that they suffer from heartburn at least once a month, you can see why antacids are so common in medicine cabinets across the country.

For many people, especially those with mild or occasional acid reflux, antacids are the only medication you'll ever need to treat your acid reflux. Most doctors will recommend continued use of antacids if they reduce your heartburn or other reflux symptoms.

Like any over-the-counter medication, it's important to discuss your antacid use with your doctor, especially if you've been taking them for more than a couple weeks.

How they work

Antacids come in a variety of over-the-counter forms. They can be liquid, chewable tablets, dissolvable tablets, foaming tablets, or chewing gum. Research has shown that liquid antacids reduce symptoms faster than other forms of antacids, but they're all very effective at neutralizing or absorbing acid.

Most of the over-the-counter antacids combine three basic salts — aluminum, magnesium, and calcium — with bicarbonate or hydroxide ions.

Antacids work in two primary forms, both of which involve the neutralization of acid. They do this because the chemicals in antacids are bases (or alkalis), which are the opposite of acids. When acids and bases are combined, they can neutralize each other. This neutralization alters the stomach's pH level and makes the stomach's contents less corrosive.

Some antacids contain alginic acid, which can help block stomach acid from surging up and irritating the esophagus. Alginate antacids possess a superpower that the standard antacids don't have. Sodium alginate is extracted from seaweed and, like the algae it's named for, forms a surface scum that floats atop your gastric contents. An alginate "raft" is a layer of polysaccharide polymer that, on contact with stomach acid, gels into a floating goo. Yummy. In theory, this means that if material rises from your stomach and regurgitates up your esophagus, it would be the alginate raft first. So, instead of attempting to neutralize all the stomach acid, the raft only neutralizes the part it's in contact with. The reflex of gastric contents, now neutral at the top where it matters, is blocked by the layer of alginate goo.

Other antacids contain simethicone and break down gas bubbles in your stomach from a bunch of tiny bubbles to one large bubble, theoretically reducing burping, which can help minimize the amount of stomach acid that gets pushed up into the esophagus. They're called *surfactants*, meaning that they break the surface tension of the gas bubbles.

What they're good for

Antacids can be a great option for people who rarely have to deal with reflux or heartburn. They're also a very effective tool in the fight against heartburn. They're generally fast acting and can provide near-immediate pain relief.

Choosing the most effective antacid to treat your specific case of acid reflux is critical. Each antacid works differently, but they're all used to restore the pH balance of the esophagus, stomach, and gastrointestinal (GI) tract. Finding out which antacid will be most effective for your reflux can be difficult, especially because there are so many different over-the-counter antacids available.

Here are just a few of the commonly used antacids on the market today:

- **Equate:** Equate is an antacid that is taken to help reduce heartburn symptoms and gas. Active ingredients include aluminum hydroxide, magnesium hydroxide, and simethicone. Avoid Equate if you have kidney disease or a magnesium-restricted diet.

- **Gaviscon:** Gaviscon is an alginic antacid that helps neutralize stomach acid while also creating that goo barrier (see the preceding section). Active ingredients include alginic acid, aluminum hydroxide, and magnesium carbonate. Check with your doctor if you have kidney disease, a history of kidney stones, or severe constipation, or if you're dehydrated.

- **Maalox:** Maalox, in liquid or tablet form, is calcium carbonate taken to temporarily neutralize acid. If you have a history of kidney stones or a parathyroid gland disorder, or if you're taking an antibiotic, avoid taking Maalox.

✔ **Milk of magnesia:** Milk of magnesia is magnesium hydroxide. It temporarily neutralizes acid. It's also used as a laxative. Some medications may interact with milk of magnesia; before using milk of magnesia, check with your doctor and pharmacist if you're taking any other medications.

✔ **Pepto-Bismol:** Pepto-Bismol is bismuth subsalicylate, and it's used for heartburn and diarrhea. Bismuth subsalicylate can pass into breast milk, so check with your doctor if you're breastfeeding.

✔ **Rolaids:** Rolaids contains calcium carbonate and magnesium hydroxide to temporarily neutralize your gastric acid.

✔ **Tums:** Tums contains calcium carbonate and is similar in function and use to Rolaids and Maalox.

Temporarily neutralizing gastric acid has the potential for *acid rebound*. Acid rebound is an increase in production of gastric acid that may occur after the initial neutralizing effect of an antacid. It's akin to your stomach saying, "Oh my gosh, that must have been a ginormous meal! Better make a ton more acid." It occurs most symptomatically when antacids containing calcium carbonate are taken.

What they're not so good for

Just because antacids are commonly used by patients with acid reflux, doesn't mean they're the most effective treatment for reflux. If you have frequent cases of reflux or gastroesophageal reflux disease (GERD), you may find antacids won't get the job done. Just like other acid neutralizers, antacids don't treat the cause of the problem — it's still the movement of the esophagus that's messed up, not an abundance of acid. Antacids simply manage pain and reduce the damage done from acid that's already made it's way into the esophagus, larynx, or mouth.

Although antacids can effectively minimize your heartburn-related discomfort, they have the potential to lead to worse problems in the future. Antacids themselves aren't particularly dangerous, but the relief they provide may prevent you from getting medical assistance to thoroughly suppress acid and prevent or heal damage and won't encourage you to be screened for Barrett's esophagus. Left untreated, even minor exposure to stomach acid can cause serious damage to your esophagus, larynx, and teeth.

Another important factor about antacids is that their effectiveness varies significantly from person to person. For some people, antacids are a miracle cure; for others, antacids have little to no impact. And this variability isn't just from person to person, it's from drug to drug. Although all antacids serve the same purpose (neutralizing acid), the exact ingredients and methodology can vary. One form of antacid may have no affect on your heartburn or other reflux symptoms, but another may be your ticket to a heartburn-free life. So, don't be afraid to try different types of over-the-counter antacids to find which formula works best for you. Just make sure you look for the active ingredient of the one that failed, so you can choose an antacid with a different chemical for round two.

Possible side effects

Every drug has potential side-effects, and these side-effects can vary based on length of use, frequency of use, and dosage. The good news is that antacids are generally quite safe, and rarely lead to long-term or high-risk health conditions. However, that doesn't mean you should consume them like a box of chocolates, even though some chewable antacids are quite tasty. If you find yourself taking antacids several times a week or daily, consult your doctor as soon as possible. It may be time for a prescription drug, or a different type of over-the-counter acid reducer.

Over-the-counter versions of prescription drugs

Some medications are made "prescription only" for several reasons. First, prescription-only drugs are typically more potent or require higher dosages. Prescription medications also tend to have the potential for more serious medical complications and side effects. Due to this increased risk, prescriptions are required to ensure the patient's safety. If a patient has to get a prescription, she'll have to check in with her doctor, who can then evaluate the effectiveness of the medication and examine her for any possible side effects.

Prescription medications require a written order from a physician, dentist, or nurse practitioner. Prescription drugs are used to treat specific medical problems. Labeling on prescription drugs undergoes more scrutiny than it does for over-the-counters. Prescription drugs come with detailed descriptions of what's in the drug, how it should be used, any potential side effects, and known drug interactions.

Over-the-counter drugs on the other hand, do not require prescriptions. They're considered medicines for conditions people are able to diagnose and treat without medical assistance (for instance, a headache or cold). Although they come with usage instructions, the amount of information about active and inactive ingredients, side effects, and drug interactions may not be as detailed or under the same level of scrutiny as it is for prescription medications. This is because most over-the-counter drugs are considered relatively safe at standard dosages in healthy patients and medical complications are unlikely. But remember, just because a medication is sold over-the-counter doesn't mean it's risk free. It's still an active drug, and all active drugs, whether prescription, over-the-counter, herbals, or your Aunt Audrey's elixir, have possible side effects.

Be sure to monitor side effects when you begin or change a treatment plan. Make sure to keep a detailed list and discuss the severity, frequency, and impact of your symptoms and side effects with your physician. A chalky aftertaste, diarrhea, or constipation are the most common side effects associated with antacids, but there are others you should be aware of. Be sure to seek medical attention if you notice any of the following:

- ✔ Bone pain
- ✔ Bloody urine
- ✔ Difficult or painful urination
- ✔ Flank pain (pain on one side of the body between the upper abdomen and the back)
- ✔ Headache
- ✔ Hives
- ✔ Mental or mood changes
- ✔ Muscle pain, weakness, or twitching
- ✔ Swelling of ankles
- ✔ Swelling of the face, lips, tongue, or throat
- ✔ Trouble breathing

Unless your doctor notices specific warning signs or you have known risk factors (such as kidney disease, heart failure, or medications that interact), your doctor probably won't recommend you stop taking antacids if they help reduce your symptoms. If you continue to follow your doctor's instructions and monitor for any associated health risks or complications, antacids can be an essential component in treating your reflux.

Reducing Acid Production

Whereas antacids help neutralize stomach acid, other medications target acid production. In some cases, your physician may recommend combining antacids with medications that reduce overall acid production, making less acid available to cause problems (instead of simply neutralizing the acid that has already splashed into the esophagus).

Although antacids are used to combat already existing symptoms, two other types of drugs are used to prevent stomach acid from being a problem in the first place: H2 receptor antagonists and proton-pump inhibitors.

H2 receptor antagonists

H2 receptor antagonists (also known as H2 blockers) are prescribed to treat occasional reflux that results from too much stomach acid making its way up the esophagus and causing esophageal inflammation.

These drugs used to be prescription only, but they've recently been approved for over-the-counter sales. The only difference between the over-the-counter and prescription forms of the drug is dosage.

It's common for an H2 receptor antagonist to be prescribed alongside other medications as part of a reflux or GERD treatment plan. Many doctors recommend using H2 receptor antagonists to help reduce the severity and frequency of acid reflux attacks, while using antacids to help alleviate the immediate symptoms associated with heartburn and reflux.

Your doctor may recommend taking antacids and H2 receptor antagonists together to prevent your reflux, but don't take them within one hour of each other. Taking antacids within the same hour can make the H2 blocker take longer to work.

How they work

H2 receptor antagonists target one of the critical components in acid reflux, stomach acid. Unlike antacids, which reduce or neutralize already existing stomach acid, H2 receptor antagonists block or prevent the production of new stomach acid. They reduce stomach acid production by blocking histamine receptors in stomach cells. *Histamine* is a neurotransmitter common in the body. In the stomach, histamine is one of the triggers for acid production. H2 blockers reduce the acidity level of the stomach, so even if the stomach's contents enter the esophagus, there is less esophageal damage and inflammation.

This type of drug can be given in one of two ways: by mouth or injection through an intravenous (IV) line. The injection version is used solely in the hospital. Generally, H2 receptor antagonists are taken orally once or twice daily. Some patients find that they only need to take the medication once a day, shortly after dinner but before bedtime.

Like other medications, your specific dose and treatment regime will be determined by your doctor, based on your symptoms as well as your reaction to the medication.

Histamine receptors are most active in the evenings, so you get more bang for your buck taking your H2 receptor antagonists toward the end of the day. Discuss the best timing with your doctor or pharmacist.

What they're good for

H2 receptor antagonists are inexpensive and can be very helpful in treating mild to moderate cases of acid reflux. Clinical trials have shown that people who only have symptoms a couple times a month respond well to this type of medication. Studies have found that around half of all GERD patients respond favorably to treatment with H2 receptor antagonists.

This type of drug can be very helpful in reducing the number and severity of symptoms associated with acid reflux. Although H2 blockers rarely eliminate every symptom, they can have a dramatic impact on your day-to-day well-being. They're most helpful when you're anticipating reflux. If you know you're going to be having a few drinks or going out to an especially spicy meal, this particular type of drug can be a great tool. Taking an H2 receptor antagonist about an hour before you go out can significantly reduce the risk of suffering an excruciating bout of heartburn or other acid reflux symptoms. However, this "as needed" dosage should be an occasional thing — don't abuse it.

Another benefit of H2 receptor antagonists is the impact they have on the esophagus. Several studies have shown that these types of drugs can help heal the damage that acid reflux does to the esophagus. Although the drug itself has been shown to speed esophageal healing, there's also the fact that these types of drugs provide longer-term relief than antacids. H2 blockers help prevent reflux flare-ups instead of simply neutralizing them as they manifest. This means fewer flares and more time for the esophagus to heal before it's exposed to corrosive stomach acid again.

What they're not so good for

Although H2 receptor antagonists can be great for about half of GERD patients, others still have breakthrough symptoms of reflux despite taking them.

H2 blockers usually provide longer relief than antacids, but they also take longer to work. While antacids can provide near immediate relief from heartburn and other reflux symptoms, H2 receptor antagonists usually take at least an hour to provide any relief. This type of medication isn't ideal for immediate flare-ups, but it's often effective for long-term acid reflux reduction and relief.

H2 blockers do provide relief for a longer period of time than antacids, but they're still a short-term fix for your reflux. They only affect stomach acid production for a short period, meaning that your body will return to its usual acid production after you stop taking the medication.

Potential side effects

Pay attention to both the frequency and severity of any side effects. Also make sure to tell your doctor about any changes to side effects that you notice. Good news: Just because you experience a side effect when you start taking a specific medication doesn't mean that you'll always have to deal with that side effect. It's common for some side effects, especially mild ones, to go away after a patient has been on a particular medication for a few weeks or even a few days.

Just like any of the other over-the-counter reflux medications, you shouldn't take H2 receptor antagonists for more than two weeks without getting the green light from your doctor. You should be aware of a variety of side effects associated with H2 blockers. For instance, constipation and diarrhea have been reported. Dizziness, headaches, nausea, and vomiting are other side effects that have been associated with H2 receptor antagonists.

Proton-pump inhibitors

Proton-pump inhibitors (PPIs) are another medication commonly prescribed for patients with acid reflux. Like H2 receptor antagonists, PPIs help prevent acid reflux outbreaks instead of treating symptoms that have already manifested.

PPIs are the most common medication prescribed to GERD patients. In fact, they're among the most widely prescribed medications in the world, with 119 million U.S. prescriptions written in 2009 alone.

This type of drug comes in both prescription and over-the-counter forms. The main difference between the over-the-counter and prescription PPIs is the dosage of the drug.

If you take an over-the-counter variety, be sure to follow the usage instructions carefully and do not take them for more than two weeks unless you have permission from your doctor.

Just like H2 receptor antagonists, PPIs are often prescribed in conjunction with antacids. PPIs help prevent and reduce future outbreaks of acid reflux, while the antacids provide immediate relief for heartburn and reflux flare-ups.

How they work

Just like H2 receptor antagonists, PPIs reduce the production of stomach acid. Both drugs block gastric or stomach acid secretion, but they do so in different ways. Instead of shutting down histamine receptors in acid-producing stomach cells like H2 receptor antagonists, PPIs disable the pumps that push acid into the stomach.

This raises the stomach's pH level, making the stomach's contents less acidic. By reducing the acidity of the stomach, there's less acid available to shoot into the esophagus. When you do experience reflux, your stomach's contents will do significantly less damage to your esophagus.

This type of drug reduces stomach acid production by blocking a particular enzyme in the wall of the stomach that is responsible for acid production. PPIs, just like the name implies, block proton pumps in your stomach. These pumps function by taking non-acidic potassium ions out of the stomach and replacing them with an acidic hydrogen ion. By pumping these hydrogen ions into the stomach, the stomach's contents become more and more acidic with hydrogen chloride, a powerful acid. PPIs block this function, reducing the amount of acidic hydrogen ions pumped into the stomach, and lowering the overall acid balance or pH.

Although there are several different PPIs, they all work in essentially the same way. Clinical research hasn't found evidence that any particular PPI medication is more effective than the others. The main differences between the various PPI drugs is their speed of action, potential drug interactions, and how they're broken down by the liver and exit your bloodstream. So, don't worry if you doctor prescribes you one particular brand, while your close friend gets another. Both drugs may be effective, but your friend may be on a medication that's known to have complications with PPIs, forcing his doctor to prescribe a different brand.

What they're good for

Just like H2 receptor antagonists, PPIs are great for preventing and reducing the severity of future acid reflux outbreaks. In fact, the acid-suppressing capability of a PPI is far greater than an H2 blocker. They're very effective tools for lowering your stomach's acid level and regulating your stomach's pH. Even when you do have a bout of reflux, PPIs can help minimize the severity of the associated symptoms. This also means that there will be less damage done to your esophagus over the long term.

That's why taking an H2 receptor antagonist or PPI can have an impact on your overall risk of developing more serious complications associated with reflux, such as esophageal stricture, Barrett's esophagus, or esophageal cancer.

Although PPIs take longer to work than antacids or H2 receptor antagonists, they generally provide longer-lasting protection. Most of the PPIs currently on the market are taken once every 24 hours. Occasionally your doctor will need to push up the dose to control your heartburn symptoms. If you have a cough, hoarseness, throat clearing, or asthma, your doctor may prescribe twice-daily PPIs from the get-go, and continue them for three months to see if you have any improvement in your symptoms.

Because they help reduce the acidity level inside the stomach, PPIs are also very helpful in reducing your risk of developing stomach and esophageal *ulcers* (shallow divots in the lining of the stomach or esophagus that can lead to discomfort and further health complications, but rarely requiring surgery). PPIs can be used to heal esophagitis. PPIs are also commonly prescribed to help treat patients diagnosed with Barrett's esophagus. There is a possibility that taking PPIs twice a day may shorten the length of your Barrett's esophagus, thus reducing the risk that it will advance to esophageal cancer.

What they're not so good for

Just like H2 receptor antagonists, PPIs take some time to begin working, but they're slower than H2s. This means they aren't ideal for treating immediate reflux flare-ups or popping before a hedonistic night on the town. They also don't treat some specific symptoms of reflux complications such as the feeling of food sticking in your throat from a stricture or narrowing of the esophagus.

PPIs can reduce the amount of acid that your esophagus, larynx, or teeth are exposed to, but they won't directly heal any previous damage. They can still be helpful, however, in that they reduce the frequency and severity of your reflux flare-ups. This gives your body more time to heal between outbreaks, and minimizes the damage done by any particular reflux outbreak. The esophagus and larynx may heal on their own when no longer exposed to acid.

PPIs can be very helpful in treating GERD over the long run, but they're not the perfect cure. Just because your symptoms are reduced, doesn't mean you can eat or drink whatever you want. One of the issues associated with PPIs is that patients who find relief may not make the necessary lifestyle changes to reduce the risks associated with acid reflux. Despite what some patients may believe, a PPI prescription is not a free pass to revert back to old habits. The reality is that you can essentially eat your way out of the protection PPIs provide.

If you take PPIs, be careful to strictly follow the usage instructions. Taken properly, PPIs will block most but not all acid from the stomach, and you can retain a healthy balance.

Potential side effects

Recent research has suggested that there are several possible side effects associated with PPIs. Some of these are the result of overuse and misuse, but there are also some serious risks associated with proper long-term use. It's fairly common for PPIs to be used to treat GERD patients. Because GERD is a chronic condition, you may end up being on some sort of medicine for much of your life.

How, when, and why does a prescription drug go over the counter?

There are a wide variety of reasons why any particular drug goes from a prescription medication to an over-the-counter version. Some of these reasons are for the patient's good; others are for the good of the drug manufacturer. For example, advertising for over-the-counter drugs have much lower standards for informing consumers about potential side effects, drug interactions, and new research. This is possible because prescription drugs are regulated by the Food and Drug Administration (FDA), while over-the-counter drugs are regulated by the U.S. Federal Trade Commission (FTC), which applies lower standards about the scientific basis of safety and efficacy. Making a drug over-the-counter can also make it easier for drug companies to get their products directly in the hands of consumers without the "interference" of doctors through direct-to-consumer advertising.

But before you start viewing over-the-counter drugs as risky cash grabs by greedy pharmaceutical companies, there are several facts to consider about the process of turning a prescription drug into an over-the-counter medication. On the positive side, being over-the-counter makes it easier for consumers to obtain the medication. If you're busy, finding time to see the doctor just to get a prescription to deal with your heartburn or reflux can be a hassle.

Whatever the reason that a particular manufacturer decides to make a drug over-the-counter instead of prescription, the process is the same. First, the drug has to qualify for over-the-counter use. Drugs are generally denied over-the-counter status if they can't be used safely without instruction or supervision, they're habit forming, or they have too great a potential for harmful side effects. In order for a drug to switch to either a prescription or over-the-counter form, it must go through the "over-the-counter drug review." This can be done through a nongovernment professional review panel that assesses the drug's success rate, as well as its risks, to determine if it should be made available over-the-counter. It can also be done by submitting a new drug application. During this process, the drug's manufacturers submit research and evidence that the drug is appropriate and safe for self-administration.

In both cases, the FDA will consider whether patients will be able to achieve the desired results without endangering their safety. If for any reason the FDA determines this isn't possible, the drug won't be allowed to be sold over-the-counter. No drug is completely safe, but the FDA's decision will be based on a risk-benefit analysis. When in doubt, the FDA will side with patient safety. This is why you can be fairly certain that your over-the-counter medication will be safe. But remember, just because it's okayed for over-the-counter use doesn't mean it isn't potentially harmful — all biologically active substances have side effects. Be sure to consult with your doctor or pharmacist when starting any over-the-counter treatment regimen, and follow the drug's usage instructions carefully.

Due to the potential side effects and risks associated with long-term use of PPIs, it's important that your doctor give you not only detailed instructions on use and dosage, but also clear recommendations for the length of treatment.

Make annual follow-up appointments with your doctor to ensure that you're not developing complications. There are a few main side effects most commonly associated with PPIs:

- ✔ **Rebound acid hyper secretion risk:** This kind of dependence on PPIs can develop after just a few weeks of use. The fact that these drugs can lead to rebound acid highlights how important following usage instructions and duration recommendations can be.

- ✔ **Osteoporosis and bone fractures:** PPIs put you at a heightened risk for these conditions, which are most commonly linked to multiple daily dose or long-term use. Generally, the spine, hip, and wrist are the most susceptible to osteoporosis and fracture from PPI use.

- ✔ **Infections:** It doesn't matter if you've been a long-term PPI user or you've just begun using the drug. Because PPIs reduce the amount of acid in the stomach, they also reduce one of the key defense systems against ingested bacterial infection. If you eat spoiled food, for example, without gastric acid the bacteria can make it through your stomach and cause disease. It's not always great to fool Mother Nature!

Each specific type of PPI may have its own drug interaction or side-effect risks. What can be a concurring interaction with one specific PPI is harmless with another. This is why it's essential for you to discuss with your pharmacist any and all pills you take, including vitamins, herbals, and over-the-counter meds.

Strengthening the Lower Esophageal Sphincter

The other drugs discussed in this chapter pertain to acid production and acid neutralization, but prokinetics focus on the lower esophageal sphincter (LES). This type of medication is aimed at addressing the root cause of acid reflux instead of simply reducing symptoms.

Prokinetics are available by prescription only and come in liquid, tablet, IV, and subcutaneous injection form. They're often used in conjunction with other acid reflux and GERD medications, such as H2 receptor antagonists and PPIs. However, the main difference with this class of drug comes down to risks. The potential side effects and complications associated with prokinetics are significantly more serious than the other generally benign acid reflux medications. Due to the potential for serious side effects, this type of drug will only be prescribed for the most severe GERD cases.

How they work

Prokinetics are a type of drug that helps strengthen the LES by increasing the pressure of the muscles in the LES. If you have acid reflux, your LES is likely the primary culprit behind your discomfort. A weakened LES allows your stomach's contents to pass back out of the stomach and into the esophagus.

By strengthening your LES, this particular class of drug can dramatically impact your reflux. In some cases, this medication can strengthen your LES to the point where it functions completely normally. This means no more reflux — food and fluid go into the stomach and stay there. Even if this drug doesn't completely eliminate your reflux, it can have a significant impact on the severity and frequency of your reflux outbursts. A stronger LES will malfunction less frequently, and will allow less stomach content to escape into the esophagus. Not only will your reflux outbursts be less frequent, but they'll generally be less painful when they do occur.

This type of medication also helps empty the stomach's contents faster. As you may know, the longer food is in your stomach, the more likely you are to experience a bit of reflux. By simply reducing the amount of time that food stays in your stomach, you reduce the likelihood that you'll suffer from heart-burn or other reflux symptoms.

Because they have a short *half-life* (the time a drug remains in your blood-stream), prokinetics are usually taken two to four times daily before meals and at bedtime.

What they're good for

This particular drug type is very good at strengthening muscles and increas-ing movement in your digestive tract. This drug will help your LES squeeze and enhance the movement of the muscular wall of your stomach and intestines, making food and fluid pass through your digestive system more quickly. When it comes to treating GERD, most physicians agree that proki-netics taken alone are comparable to H2 blockers, but slightly less effective than PPIs. To maximize their effectiveness, they're often prescribed in con-junction with acid neutralizers like H2s or PPIs.

As mentioned earlier in this section, they're also extremely effective at improving esophageal movement. These types of drugs don't just strengthen the squeeze of the muscles of the LES, they also enhance the squeeze of the muscles lining your esophagus. This makes it easier for you to swallow and for your esophagus to push any food or fluid down into the stomach, which can be helpful when you have acid reflux. Not only is it harder for acid to sneak past the LES, but it's also easier for your body to push any of your stomach's contents back down by swallowing.

With stronger movement of the gastrointestinal tract muscles, food and fluids pass through the stomach and intestines more quickly. This faster transport reduces the severity and frequency of GERD symptoms. When used in conjunction with other acid-suppressing or acid-neutralizing drugs, prokinetics can be a useful tool in managing acid reflux.

What they're not so good for

As mentioned earlier in this section, prokinetics are used only in the most extreme GERD cases due to the high risk level associated with their use. These aren't drugs you should be on if you only have mild or occasional heartburn or reflux symptoms. If your reflux is primarily associated with specific habits or your diet, this type of medication is unlikely to have any effect on your symptoms.

You shouldn't use prokinetics in an attempt to relieve or treat your immediate reflux symptoms. Unlike antacids, H2 blockers, or PPIs, prokinetics will have no direct impact on your symptoms. Instead of neutralizing acid or reducing acid production, these drugs simply target the muscles responsible for reflux. This means that taking a dose of prokinetics will have little immediate effect on your in-the-moment symptoms.

Due to the high-risk side effects associated with long-term use of prokinetics, doctors don't prescribe them lightly. Modest reflux symptoms won't get you a prescription for this drug family.

Potential side effects

Prokinetics are one of the higher-risk medications associated with the treatment of acid reflux. Due to the serious medical risks linked with long-term prokinetic use, some physicians will not even consider prokinetics as a treatment option. If they do, it tends to be only in the most severe GERD cases, and it's often done under strict supervision.

One of the most significant side effects associated with prokinetics is the development of _extrapyramidal symptoms,_ which are closely associated side effects that impact your nervous system. They include

✔ Muscle spasms

✔ Movements of the tongue and lips

✔ Slurred speech

If you find that you're experiencing any of these symptoms, stop the medication immediately and contact your doctor. Your doctor will likely recommend that you stop any prokinetic use completely. In most cases, especially when caught early, these symptoms will disappear around 24 hours after the last dose of prokinetics.

Doctors rarely prescribe prokinetic medication to patients under 20, because younger patients have a significantly higher risk for these extrapyramidal symptoms.

That's not the only thing you have to worry about when being treated with prokinetics. On top of diarrhea, nervousness, anxiousness, and agitation, there's also a heightened risk of serious cardiac arrhythmias, some of which might be fatal if not treated immediately.

Some studies have also found an increase in pituitary prolactin release, which can lead to impotence, *galactorrhea* (inappropriate milk release from the breasts, even in men), or menstrual disorders.

More alarming is when patients develop neurological disorders such as

- ✔ **Dystonia:** A neurological movement disorder where sustained muscle contractions cause twisting and repetitive movements or abnormal postures
- ✔ **Tardive dyskinesia:** A neurological disorder that leads to frequent, involuntary body movements or spasms

These disorders are extremely serious and something you'll hopefully never have to deal with. This class of drugs should be avoided in folks who already have a movement disorder, such as people with Parkinson's disease.

Because of the potential to develop these serious, sometimes incurable, side effects, doctors are always very cautious when prescribing prokinetics.

Be certain that you discuss with your doctor all the possible side effects associated with prokinetics before you begin any form of treatment involving these drugs. Make sure you're aware of all the warning signs and notify your doctor immediately at the first indication of any of the side effects.

As always, you and your doctor need to weigh the risk factors associated with this medication versus the possible benefits. That said, don't let the potential side effects scare you away from a treatment that could improve your life, especially if your doctor believes the benefits will be worth the risk.

Alternative Options: Taking a Holistic Approach

For many people, the idea of depending on medication isn't appealing. Whether you just can't afford to spend the money on a prescription or over-the-counter medication, or you don't want to be reliant on pharmaceuticals, you may find that a more holistic or naturalistic approach is appropriate.

Lifestyle and dietary changes can be an effective method to treat acid reflux and GERD. Learning which foods to avoid, what habits to break, and watching your weight are all useful tools in your battle with reflux. But they aren't the only tools at your disposal.

From old wives' tale remedies to the burgeoning field of homeopathic and natural medicine, there are treatment options outside of taking pills, getting shots, or having surgery. You may find that a holistic approach is effective for you. But don't forget that such natural or homeopathic treatments may still have potential side effects. Natural is not the same as safe.

Although this approach can be helpful, it's important to keep in contact with your doctor. She'll help you assess whether your treatment regimen is working effectively, as well as whether it's putting your health at risk. Just because you aren't taking a pharmaceutical doesn't mean there won't be complications. So, although you should be open to trying a more holistic or naturalistic approach, it's still important to understand the potential risks and evaluate the effectiveness of your treatment plan. Finally, no matter how well your chosen remedy seems to be working, it never hurts to have an examination by a doctor, just to be sure you aren't doing more harm than good.

When you're trying to find ways to handle your reflux symptoms, you may turn to the Internet to do some research. The good news: The Internet is a treasure-trove of information. The bad news: The Internet is a treasure-trove of hogwash. Just because you read something on the Internet, doesn't mean it's true. What we present in this section are some of the more popular homeopathic remedies. There is very little to no scientific evidence to back up these remedies. And as always, talk with your doctor about what you're considering before you try it.

Baking soda

You can find lots of advice about effective ways to stave off or treat reflux or heartburn, but it turns out one old standby actually has some merit. For years, patients, as well as some doctors, have been recommending baking soda to help relieve acid reflux and heartburn symptoms. (Other doctors shudder when they contemplate the huge dose of sodium you get when you ingest baking soda.)

To understand why baking soda may work, you need to understand a little bit about baking soda. As the name implies, acid reflux involves acid — stomach acid, to be specific. You may remember from seventh-grade science class when you built that bicarbonate volcano that acids and bases neutralize each other. Baking soda, or sodium bicarbonate, is alkaline. This is why consuming a small amount of baking soda can help neutralize any stomach acid that's managed to make its way into your esophagus.

The nice thing about this treatment is that it's readily available around the house. It's a common household cooking product that's okay for most people to take, as long as you don't need to monitor your sodium intake. (Check with your doctor if you're not sure.)

Baking soda won't treat the root cause of your acid reflux. Like antacids, it temporarily neutralizes the stomach acid. And it does so fast. That's one of the primary advantages of using baking soda to treat your reflux. It's fast, cheap, and available.

Most people treat reflux with baking soda by mixing ½ teaspoon to 1 teaspoon of baking soda in a glass of water. This can be very helpful for unexpected flare-ups or the occasional bout of heartburn, but it shouldn't be used as a long-term treatment. Due to its extremely high salt content, long-term use of baking soda as a form of heartburn or reflux relief can lead to side effects like swelling and nausea.

Feel free to pull out the baking soda for some quick relief of a painful explosion of heartburn, but don't expect it to be a long-term treatment or solution. And if you have issues with sodium, like high blood pressure, kidney disease, or congestive heart failure, definitely check with your doctor first.

If you're using baking soda as a heartburn remedy for more than two weeks, consult your doctor.

Acid neutralizers

Acid neutralizers are among the more common ways people treat their heartburn and acid reflux. Antacids are the most common type of acid neutralizers. The good news, if you want to take a holistic approach, is that it's possible to make your own acid-neutralizing medications at home. Whether these work is up for debate.

Aside from getting some of the chemical compounds used commonly in antacids, such as calcium carbonate, there are other common home remedies. One of the most popular self-care remedies is to drink about 1 ounce of apple cider vinegar. Most physicians question the validity of using a weak acid to treat heartburn and reflux. That said, there are enough people who swear by it as an effective tool that it may be worth trying. That's up to you.

Aside from apple cider vinegar, aloe vera and coconut water have also been touted as great home remedies for heartburn and reflux, but as with apple cider vinegar, there is little to no scientific data to confirm their effectiveness.

Whether they're homemade or store bought, acid neutralizers do exactly what the name says: They help to neutralize acid. This makes the pH higher, or more neutral, which means the stomach contents will do less damage to any tissue they're exposed to. As noted, this type of treatment doesn't solve the cause of your reflux, but it may help minimize the damage and manage the pain.

This type of treatment is especially helpful for people who suffer from severe bouts of heartburn. By neutralizing the acid in the esophagus, the burn goes away. Even more significantly, neutralization reduces the amount of esophageal damage that acid can do. As the acid is neutralized, it becomes less potent, which means it'll be less corrosive and do significantly less damage to your esophagus, larynx, or teeth.

However, acid neutralizers only offer temporary relief. They begin working almost as soon as you take them, but the relief is only short term and it'll do nothing to prevent future flare-ups. Because acid neutralizers work by altering the pH balance in your esophagus and stomach, your body quickly reacts by increasing acid secretion.

There are benefits to treating your acid reflux with acid neutralizers. First, they're readily available. They're also quite inexpensive compared to most other medical treatments. Another big advantage is the speed at which they provide relief. Other medications and remedies can help reduce outbreaks and relieve symptoms, but none of them is as able to relieve immediate symptoms with the same speed and efficiency.

Most important, they're generally quite safe. Unless you overuse or abuse them, there are very few side effects associated with their use.

The main problem with acid neutralizers is that they don't do anything to address the cause of your reflux, and they don't suppress acid all the time, just when you take them. Although taking an acid neutralizer before a meal can help stave off heartburn, it's not going to stop your acid reflux. Instead it's simply neutralizing the acid that is pushed into your esophagus by your reflux, before you begin to experience any pain. The neutralizer can help provide immediate relief for current or imminent symptoms, but it won't help you with the long-term management of your reflux.

You'll also need to be careful not to overuse acid neutralizers.

They won't neutralize all the acid in your stomach, but they can neutralize enough to reduce your body's ability to destroy and fight bacteria you ingest. This can lead to illness and infection. So, don't hesitate to use acid neutralizers to treat your reflux, especially for immediate or short-term symptoms, but don't rely on them to make all your reflux troubles disappear.

Herbal remedies

Naturopathic medicine is one of the fastest-growing industries in the medical field. Part of this growth is due to dissatisfaction with the rising cost of medical care and pharmaceuticals. And maybe if these naturopathic and homeopathic treatments weren't effective, people wouldn't continue to use them. However, there is little scientific data on their effectiveness.

There is a wide variety of possible herbal remedies, and some are more common than others. The first is using ginger tea to help relieve heartburn and minimize acid reflux flare-ups.

The next time you have a bout of heartburn, try adding a teaspoon of gingerroot to a cup of boiling water and let it steep for ten minutes or so. Strain the ginger out of the water before you drink it. Just like many of the acid neutralizers, this particular remedy works quickly — some people claim nearly immediate reduction of symptoms. Chamomile, mint, or fenugreek tea have also been recommended for reducing acid reflux symptoms.

Some dietitians believe that fenugreek seeds can be an effective treatment against heartburn and reflux as well. One or two teaspoons added to your food may help coat the lining of your stomach, making it more difficult for acid to move up your esophagus. The seeds may also help prevent inflammation and damage to your stomach, which may help reduce your risk for stomach ulcers. Some dietitians believe that herbal supplements like slippery elm have also been shown to soothe the digestive tract and help reduce heartburn and acid reflux attacks. Again, the scientific community has not proven this, so try at your own risk.

Even just a cursory search of the Internet will generate hundreds of potential herbal remedies. Feel free to consult with a naturopathic physician about your symptoms and any possible treatments they suggest.

Note: As your health advocate, your doctor will likely point out the lack of scientific study on safety and efficacy for these herbal remedies.

Naturopathic physicians are not recognized as doctors in most states. This means they may not have been rigorously trained, and don't have to pass testing, be licensed by the state, have continuing training requirements, or be subject to the oversight of a state medical review board like your regular doctor. This doesn't mean that they can't be trusted to provide effective and safe care, but it does mean that you should carefully vet your naturopathic physician. And remember that it never hurts to get a second opinion from a licensed medical professional.

Digestive enzymes

Some people who suffer from chronic acid reflux may be able to find relief by taking digestive enzymes. However, published, peer-reviewed studies are lacking to prove that digestive enzymes can be effective in dealing with symptoms associated with acid reflux while also improving overall digestive health. The recommendations for the specific mix of digestive enzymes to try varies from case to case. A homeopathic specialist may help guide you to a homeopathic method for treating your reflux.

Usually a homeopathic specialist will want to develop digestive enzymes specifically for you. He'll develop these digestive compounds based on the specifics of your case and your symptoms. The two most commonly used ingredients in these homemade digestive enzymes are slippery elm and licorice root. These enzymes can be effective, but your homeopathic specialist will most likely suggest making lifestyle changes as well. These generally include monitoring your diet, reducing your fat intake, reducing your alcohol intake, and minimizing caffeine consumption.

One key thing to note about digestive enzymes is that they aren't immediate cures. If you have a severe case of heartburn kicking in, taking a digestive enzyme compound created by your homeopathic specialist isn't likely to stop the pain.

Chewing gum

If you deal with the searing pain and discomfort associated with acid reflux and GERD, the idea that something as simple as chewing gum could help cure your reflux may seem preposterous. However, there is increasing evidence that this just may be the case. But how does it work?

First, chewing gum helps with the production of saliva. Saliva can play a critical role in helping clear acid from the esophagus, throat, and larynx. The more saliva you produce, the more you'll swallow, which will make it harder for acid to work its way up the esophagus. On top of that, the alkaline nature of saliva helps neutralize any acid it comes into contact with.

The acid-neutralizing capability of saliva is important. Several studies have found that patients who chewed gum after a meal had significantly lower acid levels than those who didn't chew gum. Less acid means less chance for reflux. It also means that symptoms like heartburn will be much less severe as the corrosive and damaging affects of regular stomach acid are reduced by the acid-neutralizing capabilities of saliva.

No one is going to suggest that chewing gum should be the only way you treat your acid reflux. But it can be a helpful and inexpensive tool to help you deal with reflux symptoms. Chewing gum after a big meal can help reduce your risk of reflux, minimize the amount of damage that a bout of reflux can do. Plus, it'll freshen your breath.

Natural licorice

Licorice is another natural remedy for acid reflux that's been widely touted by homeopathic physicians. Licorice or licorice extract is commonly used by homeopathic practitioners to treat digestive system complaints such as stomach ulcers, heartburn, colic, and *chronic gastritis* (an ongoing inflammation of the lining of the stomach). It's been used to help relieve sore throats and coughs, both of which can be symptoms of acid reflux.

Generally, licorice will be combined with several other herbs when it's used in the treatment of acid reflux. The most common herbs that are combined with licorice to treat reflux include angelica, caraway, celandine, clown's mustard plant, German chamomile, lemon balm, milk thistle, and peppermint leaf. Just like digestive enzymes, the exact combination of ingredients will depend on your specific case.

Licorice contains a substance called glycyrrhizic acid, which has been linked to headaches, swelling, sodium retention, loss of potassium, and high blood pressure, so it may not be as safe as you assume it will be. There are no peer-reviewed medical articles supporting licorice use for reflux.

If you decide you want to try licorice, look for deglycyrrhizinated licorice (DGL).

Too much of anything can be dangerous. Eating a little licorice daily won't do much harm, but eating a half pound of the stuff every day will likely lead to some problems, even if it's only black teeth and bowel movements.

Taking Your Complaint to the Doctor

With acid reflux and GERD being such common conditions, it can be difficult to decide when to seek medical treatment. You'll obviously want to seek treatment if you notice serious symptoms like difficulty swallowing, trouble breathing, or severe chest pain, but a little heartburn a few times a week may not seem worth a trip to the doctor. However, you shouldn't be afraid to consult your physician, especially when it comes to heartburn and acid reflux.

Sometimes seeking treatment for your reflux before it becomes a big problem can save you a world of hurt down the road. Whether you make an appointment with a gastroenterologist or consult your family doctor, discussing your reflux and symptoms is important. A doctor can help figure out the best method to treat your specific symptoms and educate you about the potential side effects associated with the treatment. She can also inform you about the long-term risks associated with not treating your reflux.

Finding the right doctor

When you've made the decision to seek professional help, it can be a challenge figuring out the next step: Who should I see? There are a variety of medical professionals out there who can help you with your acid reflux. You have to decide whether you want to see a general practitioner, a specialist, or even a naturopath. Any one of them may be able to assist you in cutting acid reflux out of your life.

Some of these decisions will be easier than others. If you won't even consider medication to treat your reflux symptoms, seeing your regular doctor or a specialist may not be the best option. Other times, it won't be personal preference that limits your choices, but finances. Most insurance plans cover an annual wellness exam, where you can discuss your reflux symptoms and treatments with your general practitioner. Seeing a gastroenterologist generally requires a referral from your primary-care doctor, before your insurance company will agree to pay. This is so that basic lifestyle and diet alterations, and basic reflux medications have been tried before a round of expensive and not-always-fun testing begins.

When you've made the decision to seek professional help for your reflux and decided what type of physician you're going to see, the next step is finding the right professional. With many doctors and naturopaths to choose from, finding the right one can be a daunting task.

Asking friends and associates for recommendations

Start with your friends and family. They can be extremely helpful in matching you up with the appropriate doctor despite not necessarily knowing your medical history.

One of the most important factors in selecting your doctor should be choosing someone you feel comfortable with. If you don't feel comfortable with your doctor, you won't be as honest and forthcoming about your symptoms. Consider word of mouth from loved ones. Your friends and family may not be able to assess the medical qualification of any given physician, but they do generally know you. They know the types of people you'll feel comfortable around and can often make great suggestions for physicians who fit your personality.

Generally, you can trust your friends and family to give you an honest assessment of their experience with different doctors.

Pay special attention to friends and family members who have dealt with acid reflux themselves. If you find that most of your friends and family are seeing the same physician, it may be a sign that he's the doctor for you.

Finding a specialist can often be a bit more challenging than a general practitioner or family doc. If you already have a primary-care doctor you trust, she can be very helpful in recommending a qualified specialist.

Turning to the Internet for referrals

Friends and family can offer trustworthy reviews of physicians and specialists they've seen, and the Internet can also be a useful tool. Numerous websites can help you locate doctors in your area. You can search for them by name, location, or specialty to help you narrow your search. Many of these sites also contain brief profiles of physicians where you can learn information about their specialty, how long they've been practicing, where they got their degrees, and their previous work histories.

Some of these sites are reliable and helpful. Not only can you locate doctors in your area, but you can also read reviews from previous patients. Online reviews are not as trustworthy as the recommendation or review of a friend, but seeing a large number of positive or negative reviews will give you a pretty good indication of concerns about the doctor.

Just keep in mind that the folks with negative feedback are generally the ones who flock to those sites, and the doctor isn't allowed to respond in any way due to privacy laws.

Before and after your appointment

Going to the doctor can be intimidating. Even if you're completely healthy, it's common to feel anxiety and uncertainty when you step into the doctor's office, and you forget all your questions and concerns. It's so common, that doctors even have a term for it: *white-coat syndrome.*

The first step is being prepared. You probably won't be able to completely remove any anxiety associated with going to the doctor, but being aware and ready for what's coming can alleviate some of the tension.

Being on top of your health history

The first thing any physician is going to want to look at is your medical history. This is why it's important to keep a copy of your medical records, especially if you end up switching doctors some time down the line. This information will provide essential insights into your current condition and any past health issues that may have an impact on your treatment.

The more detailed your health history is, the better the picture your doctor will have of your overall health. This will allow her to get an overview of your health and to spot any patterns or trends of concern.

Your health history should contain as much information as possible about any conditions or medical problems that immediate blood relatives have suffered, as well as any conditions, hospitalization, diseases, or surgeries you've gone through. Even if you don't know the exact medical terminology, simply describing your condition and the treatment will generally be enough to give your doctor a solid picture of your health concerns.

You'll also want to list any prescription or over-the-counter medications, herbals, holistic remedies, or vitamins that you've taken recently, as well as everything you've tried and discarded for your current symptoms. Be as specific as possible and try to include the drug name, the dosage amount, and how often you took the medication. The more information you provide your doctor, the better the chances that she'll be able to effectively treat you.

How to prep for your visit

Before your appointment, jot down a list of questions you have for your doctor — and add to that list in the days leading up to the appointment, as necessary. It's easy to forget the questions you were going to ask when you're sitting on the exam table.

Keep a short journal — two weeks should be long enough — of your daily routine. List all the times you experience reflux and all the associated symptoms. Be sure to describe the timing, length, strength, and frequency of your symptoms. Use a 1- to 10-point scale to rate your pain and other symptoms, where 1 is minor discomfort and 10 is a nuclear test going off in your chest.

When it comes to acid reflux, lifestyle and dietary choices often play a significant role. That's why it's important to keep a food and exercise journal as well. This type of journal can be compared with your reflux journal to see if any dietary or lifestyle choices are influencing or affecting your reflux. Be sure to review both before you go to your doctor, and don't hesitate to bring up any observations or questions you have regarding your journals.

When you go for your first appointment, consider brining a friend to listen along and make sure you hear and remember what the doctor says. Doctors have a lot to cover in that first appointment, and it can be rushed. If you don't have an available friend, bring a tape recorder or record the conversation about the diagnosis and treatment plans on your cellphone.

Doctor's orders: Following up

Follow-up care is essential for safe and effective treatment. Make sure to go to all appointments, and don't hesitate to call your doctor if you notice any new symptoms or issues. Depending on how your appointment goes, your physician may request a follow-up visit. Even if he doesn't ask you to come back in, he may want you to call and report any changes to your condition. This is especially true when you're starting a new treatment.

If your doctor starts you on a new medication or requests that you make some lifestyle changes in order to manage your acid reflux, checking back in can be essential. First, assuming you followed the doctor's recommendations, it'll provide him with some insight into whether the treatment is working. If he finds that it isn't helping or is actually making things worse, checking back in will give him a chance to alter your treatment so it'll be more effective. It can also help him head off any dangerous, unwanted side effects.

If you haven't been following the doctor's orders, it'll still give him helpful insight into the best way to treat your reflux. Say, for instance, that your doctor tells you to avoid spicy foods and stop drinking alcohol, but you don't abide. If your doctor knows that you can't or won't try one specific treatment, he can come up with alternative treatments, or at the very least warn you of the consequences of failing to follow his recommendations.

Either way, checking back in with your doctor after your appointment will provide him with valuable information about the effectiveness of the proposed treatment and alert him to any complications before they become serious or life threatening.

Part II
Making Diet and Lifestyle Changes

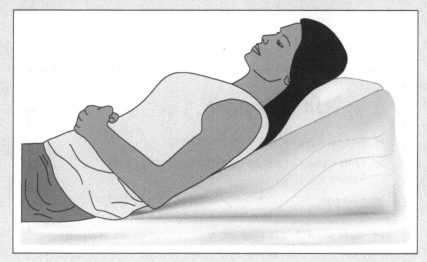

© John Wiley & Sons, Inc.

web extras

Find out more about exercising to reduce reflux in an article at www.dummies.com/extras/acidrefluxdiet.

In this part . . .

✔ Find out if you're ready to make a change.

✔ Explain your diet and lifestyle updates to family and friends.

✔ Give your kitchen a makeover to support the acid reflux diet.

✔ Make some lifestyle changes, such as sleeping in a new position and exercising more or in a different way.

Chapter 6

Getting Started on the Acid Reflux Diet

. . . .

In This Chapter

▶ Knowing when you're ready to make a change

▶ Understanding how to transition to an acid reflux diet

▶ Finding your acid reflux triggers

▶ Ridding your kitchen of the wrong foods and filling it with the right ones

▶ Considering how you cook when you have acid reflux

. . . .

Change, oh no! Starting a new plan can be scary, especially when that plan involves something as important as food. But this chapter gets you off to a good start. A pleasant transition is, well, pleasant, and it helps you stick with the diet. Maybe you feel anxious now, but when you get used to the new plan and your symptoms decrease, you'll be glad you started!

You know what they say about a journey of a thousand miles: It begins with a single step. Acknowledging that you have acid reflux was your first step in getting rid of it. See, you've already taken a whole step! Deciding you want to change it is the second step. Buying this book was a great third step, and reading it is a fourth. That's four whole steps you've taken!

Let's take a moment to revisit Step 2. Are you still feeling motivated to change your diet and some lifestyle factors, or are you wavering? It's normal to go back and forth a little when embarking on a new path. If you're certain that you want to make changes, skip the first section of this chapter and blaze right into the second section. If you're still on the fence, the first section may help you decide whether you're in or out.

You may not be ready to follow the whole plan, but you want to follow some of it. That's much better than doing nothing! Your results won't be as conclusive as if you follow the plan to a tee, but you'll probably still see some results.

When Enough Is Enough: Deciding to Make a Change

How do you know when you're ready to make changes to get rid of your acid reflux? When you answer yes to each of the following questions:

- Do you have acid reflux?
- Do you have acid reflux more than a few times a year?
- Is your acid reflux annoying or worse?
- If you had to make some changes for the rest of your life that felt a little uncomfortable or annoying, mostly at first, but those changes made your acid reflux decrease or go away, would you make those changes?

Maybe you're not certain. Maybe you think your acid reflux isn't quite bad enough to make you cut back on caffeine or red meat or those midnight snacks. If you're not ready to make changes, you're not ready. No shame in that. This book will be waiting for you when you are.

It's strange what we get used to in life. When something unusual happens, we often ignore it, even if ignoring it can cause major consequences. Such is the case with acid reflux. Maybe yours started as an annual occurrence and wasn't all that bad. Maybe you felt uncomfortable for ten minutes and then drifted off to peaceful slumber, never to think of acid reflux again until the next Thanksgiving.

But then the acid reflux began appearing monthly, and with increasing intensity. And then weekly, and then it almost seemed normal, one more unpleasant detail of life better left ignored, like traffic. Then the proverbial dam breaks and you realize that something needs to be done.

For many people, the proverbial dam break is when the antacids they've been popping like Pez stop working. Whatever that breaking point is for you, that's when you'll decide you need to make a change. Your next step will be to tell family and friends about the new diet you're starting. If you're all in, we recommend you explain the diet at least to the people who share your home and/or meals. In this section, we give you some tips for doing exactly that.

How to tell people you're close to and see often

Ask if you can talk with them. You can talk to people one on one, or in a group (for instance, your whole family at once). Once you have them all together, follow these steps:

1. If they don't already know, tell them that you have acid reflux. If necessary, tell them what acid reflux is.

2. Explain how the acid reflux negatively impacts your life.

3. Say that you want to better manage your acid reflux and that diet is going to be part of it.

4. Tell them the main foods you'll be avoiding and the main foods you'll be including.

5. Explain that you'll be eating smaller portions and not late at night. Briefly explain any other parts of your plan (for example, exercising or losing weight).

6. Tell them that this will all be easier if you have their support. Explain that supporting you is very easy.

   All they have to do is not make fun of you or your diet, and refrain from offering you the foods that give you acid reflux.

7. Ask if they would like to eat the same meals you'll be eating.

   If they show some interest or at least openness to the possibility, share some of the recipes you intend to make.

8. Warn them that you may be a little cranky when you first give up some foods you particularly like.

Taking the bull by the horns

People have a huge range of opinions about food, and some are very vocal about those opinions. Most won't even notice or care that you're on a new food plan, but some may notice and have a negative attitude or tell you information that conflicts with what's in this book or what your doctor says.

There are all kinds of theories about what works for acid reflux, just as there are theories about how to cure the hiccups. They don't all work, but people share them anyway.

Want to avoid those opinions? Then you may decide that you don't want to tell anyone about your diet, except people who cook or buy groceries with you. That's totally acceptable. For other people, sharing news about the diet will be helpful. Why? Because starting something new can make you feel vulnerable — especially if you're surrounded by opinionated people — and explaining the diet lets you frame it.

If you're surrounded by such people and you just know they'll point out the changes you're making, we recommend that you take an assertive role and tell them about your diet before they tell you. If you're assertive, you set the tone and you're in charge.

Choose what level you'd like to share your process going forward. Do you want to bring your kids grocery shopping with you? Do you want your roommate, husband, wife, or partner to cook most of the recipes? Do you want to share your progress with the people close to you? Or do you want to tell people what you're doing one time and then clam up about it? It's up to you!

How to tell colleagues and associates

You don't have to tell colleagues and associates much of anything unless you want to. If you're not sure whether to say anything, ask yourself:

- Will they notice?
- Do they care?
- Will it make life easier or harder (or no different at all) if Bob from accounting knows about your new diet?

If Bob doesn't really have much to do with you, or if he won't even notice when you order something slightly different next time you go out for lunch, you can probably keep it to yourself. On the other hand, if Bob is your close work buddy and would be a great source of support, maybe it's worth filling him in.

If you decide that you'd like to tell a colleague or other associate, follow these steps:

1. **Tell them, "I have acid reflux and I'm trying to get rid of it. I'm following a new diet and will be eating more of _____ and less of _____."**

   Most people will say, "Okay, sounds good." If they don't really care more than that, the conversation is over.

2. **If they have questions, answer them if you feel like it.**

   If you don't feel like answering their questions or you don't know the answers, say, "This is all I know at this point. I'll keep you posted."

You get to choose whether to keep them posted. This is your diet and your life, and you can share what you want and stay quiet when you want.

Transitioning to an Acid Reflux Diet

To reduce your acid reflux, you need to cut back on or give up the foods listed in Chapter 4. The variable is that you can choose the pace. Here are your options:

- ✔ **Go cold turkey.** Give up all trigger foods and do the diet 100 percent right from the beginning.
- ✔ **Ramp up slowly.** Cut out trigger foods gradually over time.

Either way, before you know it you'll avoid trigger foods without even realizing it — the plan will become easy and instinctive. But you should still decide which option works best for you. In this section, we give you some more information to help you decide.

Going cold turkey

Dive in head first!

You're in this!

Heck yeah, let's do it!

If those sentences excite you or you relate to them, your best route is cold turkey. Everyone is different. If you tend toward making big changes all at once, you'll probably do well by following this diet and plan to a tee — no messing around, no exceptions — for a month and then rating how you feel.

Normally it's wise to take change slowly, but in this case, the diet is so nuanced and easy to incorporate that we suggest taking the plunge and going cold turkey off trigger foods. This option will also give you a clearer idea of whether the diet is working for you. For instance, let's say you have acid reflux three days a week and you avoid all trigger foods for one month. If, in that month, you find that you only had acid reflux once and in the very beginning of the trial, that's a clear indicator that the diet is working for you.

Here's how to go cold turkey:

1. **Tell your friends and family about the diet, if you want.**

   After you tell them, start the diet soon after. This will keep the momentum going.

2. **Throw out trigger foods that you have in your house, if they tempt you.**

   If canned tomatoes are easy for you to ignore, keep them. If you can't possibly ignore the fresh grapefruit juice your neighbor brought over, get rid of it or ask someone else to consume it for you.

   For more on how to manage your cupboards, see the section "Giving your kitchen a makeover to support the acid reflux diet" later in this chapter.

3. **Make your meal plans and shopping list for the next week, or maybe the whole month.**

   On this cold-turkey route, you're going to do things even if you're uncomfortable with them. For instance, if you're used to a nightcap every evening before you go to bed, that's just going to have to change, at least for a month while you see what bothers your reflux and what doesn't.

4. **Decide what day and hour you're starting the diet.**

   Starting on that day and hour, you will not consume a single trigger food. Not even a teaspoon of it. Not even a small glass of orange juice. No hot sauce on your burrito. Try to stick with this for an entire month and see how you feel.

5. **Start making recipes from this book.**

   Everything you eat for one month needs to be from this book, or be another recipe or food that doesn't include any trigger foods.

Take note of how you feel as you make these changes.

Easing in

Here's the upside to easing in: It's less scary and less dramatic. Also, sometimes when we make changes slowly, they stick better. Easing in to this diet means that you still have some of the trigger foods, but maybe smaller portions of them. It could also mean that you completely cut out some trigger foods, but not others.

You may be worried that a cold-turkey approach could cause you to eliminate foods that don't trigger acid reflux in your particular case. For instance, maybe you love salsa and you don't want to give that up if you don't have to. In this situation, you may prefer the nine-day challenge, in the next section. This challenge has you eliminate trigger foods systematically and then reintroduce them.

Again, our suggestion is to go cold turkey, which means following the plan morning, noon, and night from day 1. But some progress is better than no progress, so either way, cold turkey or easing in, you're in much better shape than if you do nothing.

Taking the Nine-Day Challenge: Finding Your Acid Reflux Triggers

We don't want you to have to give up foods that you like if they don't cause problems for you. And likewise, we want you to know what foods do cause you problems so you can stay away them. Take this nine-day challenge to find out which foods bother you and which foods don't.

Cutting down or cutting out favorite foods can be tough. Some foods feel addictive, and if one of these addictive foods strikes your fancy, you may feel anxiety about waving goodbye to it. Or maybe you won't even know you're addicted to that food until you try to get rid of it.

For example, chocolate is high in fat, and that's part of why it activates acid reflux. Does this mean you can never have chocolate again? Not necessarily. You can work on cutting down, instead of cutting out. Try this nine-day challenge, and if you find out that say, chocolate, is a trigger food for you, cut it out of your life for a month to be sure. Then reintroduce small amounts of chocolate after the month-long trial.

Of course, chocolate isn't the only trigger food you may crave. Does spice and heat get you fired up in a good way (until it fires up your throat in a bad way)? If you're going cold turkey from trigger foods, you'll have to cut out all the spice and heat from your diet. It will take about a month before you know for sure whether you're better off without spice and heat. After the first month, you may be able to tolerate small portions of the trigger foods later on, especially if you eat them earlier in the day.

Before you start the challenge, journal how you feel for six whole days. Here are some questions to ask yourself:

✔ **How many times have I had acid reflux these six days?**

✔ **How bad has my acid reflux been each time I had it?** For each episode in the last six days, rate the reflux as one of the following:

- 5: The worst I've ever had

- 4: Pretty bad

- 3: Average for me

- 2: Not as bad as usual

- 1: Not a big deal at all — barely noticeable

✔ **Overall, how have I felt each of these six days?** Come up with a number for each day:

- 1: Great

- 2: Good

- 3: Fair
- 4: Bad

Add up your numbers for the whole six days. That's the number you'll compare to what you rack up in the upcoming nine-day challenge. The higher the number, the worse your reflux is.

Days 1–3: Cutting out possible culprits

The first three days require you to get rid of some things you may really like. We're sorry — but remember: If you find that those foods or beverages don't bother you when you reintroduce them (later in the trial), you can still have them!

Here are the foods to cut out the first three days:

- ✔ Alcohol
- ✔ Caffeine
- ✔ Canned foods
- ✔ Chocolate
- ✔ Citrus
- ✔ Cranberries
- ✔ Mint
- ✔ Raw garlic
- ✔ Raw onion
- ✔ Red meat
- ✔ Tomatoes

Also cut out these spices:

- ✔ Black pepper
- ✔ Cayenne
- ✔ Chili
- ✔ Curry
- ✔ Mustard
- ✔ Nutmeg

And sorry, but the list doesn't end there. (We know. "Booooo!") You'll also need to cut out:

- ✔ Carbonated beverages
- ✔ Complicated meals with lots of acidic ingredients (according to some nutritionists)
- ✔ Fried foods
- ✔ Spicy foods
- ✔ Excess fat (like butter, excess oils, and chicken skins)
- ✔ Large meals

This entire challenge, don't eat to the point of being very full. Eat just until you're satisfied, and then stop. Eating too much food at once is a big trigger of acid reflux.

And you'll also need to cut out water and air. Just kidding! Really, these lists are all you need to cut out. And it's only for a little while, so don't worry! To find out more about those trigger foods, including why they're harmful to acid reflux sufferers, read Chapter 4.

The food you may be most worried about cutting out is red meat, unless you're a vegetarian. If you're worried about cutting out red meat, just cut out fatty portions of red meat, such as burgers sizzling in grease, and have very lean versions instead. Lean protein, such as chicken and seafood, empties the stomach much quicker so it doesn't trigger acid reflux like a hamburger or a big portion of bacon might.

Days 4–6: Monitoring how you feel

All right, you cut out a lot of foods. It was only for three days, but it may have been challenging anyway. Now it's time to keep those foods away a little longer (just three more days).

Record how you feel each day. Ask yourself the same questions you asked in the six-day pre-challenge period:

- ✔ **How many times have I had acid reflux these six days?**
- ✔ **How bad has my acid reflux been each time I had it?** For each time in the last six days, rate the reflux as one of the following:
    - 5: The worst I've ever had
    - 4: Pretty bad
    - 3: Average for me

- 2: Not as bad as usual
- 1: Not a big deal at all — barely noticeable

✔ Overall, how have I felt each of these six days? Come up with a number for each day:

- 1: Great
- 2: Good
- 3: Fair
- 4: Bad

Add up your numbers for the whole six days, for each category. Compare it to your number from the six-day pre-challenge period. The higher the number, the worse your reflux is and the worse you're feeling overall. If your numbers have improved, the diet very well may be working for you.

Days 7–9: Reintroducing foods

Now, this is the fun part! The foods you missed the most can come back into your life at this point. Don't go hog wild, though. For instance, it might not be a good idea to go to a salsa festival and visit every booth if tomato, garlic, and onion turn out to be three of your triggers.

Make a list of the possible trigger foods you missed the most, and then try each of them during this three-day period. Try to have only one a day, so that it's more clear which ones, if any, are the culprit if your reflux comes back.

If you have more than three trigger foods that you very much missed, extend this part of the trial as long as needed until you identify which foods bother you and which foods don't.

Giving Your Kitchen an Acid Reflux Makeover

Renovating your cabinet contents is way easier than renovating a kitchen. But there still may be some uncomfortable moments.

If you're the type who hates to throw away food (more power to you, by the way — sustainability is the way to go), then give the food away to neighbors, friends, family, or food banks.

This part of the diet isn't just about getting rid of foods — it's also about moving the right foods in.

Cleaning your pantry

Out of sight, out of mind, so either hide those trigger foods or get rid of them. If there's a trigger food that you don't particularly like, you'll probably be fine having it in the house, even smack in the front of your pantry. Heck, if a bag of onions isn't tempting, it isn't tempting. And if onions don't trigger your reflux anyway, you can for sure keep those onions around. But if your reflux is triggered by chocolate and you love chocolate, then that economy-size bag of Lindt truffles that your Aunt Selma gave you for Christmas will need to find a new home.

If any of the items on this list tempt you, either move them to where you can't see them as easily, or get rid of them:

- Alcohol
- Black pepper
- Caffeinated coffee
- Caffeinated tea
- Canned foods
- Cayenne
- Chili powder
- Chocolate
- Citrus
- Cranberry
- Curry
- Meat (particularly red meat)
- Mint
- Mustard
- Nutmeg
- Raw garlic
- Raw onion
- Tomatoes

Stocking up on the right foods

All right, here's the direction we want to go: adding, instead of depriving. Unless you hate one of the foods in this section, add all of them to your pantry, fridge, and freezer before you start the acid reflux diet.

Bananas

Well, you just know these suckers are healthy. Many fruits are high in acid and, therefore, bad for reflux sufferers, but bananas are quite tame. And they have all these lovely nutrients:

- ✓ Fiber
- ✓ Folate
- ✓ Iron
- ✓ Magnesium
- ✓ Manganese
- ✓ Niacin
- ✓ Potassium
- ✓ Riboflavin
- ✓ Vitamin A
- ✓ Vitamin B6
- ✓ Vitamin C

One medium banana only has 110 calories and 1 gram of protein. Bananas have no cholesterol and no sodium. They're high in potassium — and healthy levels of potassium can reduce blood pressure and reduce risk of stroke. Potassium also preserves bone mineral density, reduces the chance of kidney stone formation, and protects against muscle loss.

Bananas contain the amino acid tryptophan, which helps preserve memory and also boosts mood.

On a less-appetizing note, bananas can help treat diarrhea. First, they promote regularity. Plus, the electrolytes in bananas help restore the electrolytes that are lost during a bout of diarrhea.

The easiest way to get more bananas in your diet is to just eat a banana. They're all ready to go in their own little packaging. Bananas are available year-round, and they ripen even after they're picked, unlike a strawberry. So, don't be afraid of a buying a banana that's a little green. To ripen the fruit faster, leave it out of the refrigerator or put it in the sun. The fastest way to ripen a banana is to put it in a brown paper bag, and then put that wrapped banana in the sun. If it gets overripe, peel it, freeze it, and use it in a smoothie or for baking.

If you want a healthy, natural way to replace fat in a baked recipe, use the equivalent amount of mashed banana. Bananas also make a great addition to smoothies, oatmeal, or cereal.

Fennel

Fennel root isn't a food that most people are used to eating regularly. However, it's easy to incorporate in recipes, such as soups, stir-fries, and assortments of roasted vegetables.

Fennel is a perennial, nice-smelling herb that has yellow flowers. In root form, it looks a little like a cross between celery, an onion, and a turnip (see Figure 6-1 for fennel in root form, and fennel as a dried seed).

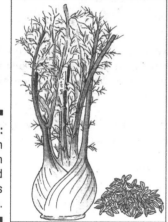

Figure 6-1:
Fennel in root form (left) and seeds (right).

Illustration by Elizabeth Kurtzman

Dried fennel seeds are often used in cooking. They have a flavor similar to anise. Fennel is great for warding off digestive problems such as heartburn (ahem), gas, bloating, and colic. Fennel may even soothe the coughing associated with acid reflux.

Leafy greens

Leafy greens are very mild on the pH scale, and that makes them a big yes for people who don't want acid reflux. Plus, not a big surprise: Eating leafy greens is good for you in general. Sure, you've known this pretty much forever, but you may not have cared enough to eat those leafy greens if your parents' idea of cooking them was to boil spinach into mushy submission.

Leafy greens are much tastier when they're not boiled. Steamed or raw is usually the most appealing route. If you're looking for the healthiest route, go for raw.

Some leafy greens include

- ✔ Broccoli
- ✔ Kale
- ✔ Lettuce
- ✔ Spinach
- ✔ Turnip greens

Leafy greens promote intestinal health and strong immune systems. All of them are healthy, but kale may be the best. This underrated green contains calcium, folate, potassium, and vitamins A, C, and K.

So, eat up on those greens — the darker the better!

Melons

Melons originated in Africa and southwest Asia, and first appeared in Europe around the end of the Roman Empire. European settlers in the New World grew honeydew and casaba melons, and Native Americans in New Mexico grew (and still grow) their own melon *cultivars* (varieties).

Like bananas, melons are very mild because they're pH friendly (more on the pH scale at the end of this chapter). That mildness makes them soothing.

Cutting a melon is easy. Just follow these steps:

1. **Wash the cantaloupe.**

   Scrub the outside of the melon with dish soap. At the very least, this will get dirt off the rind and make for a cleaner melon when you cut it. At the most, washing the outside of the melon will make you less likely to get the bacteria that the rind may be harboring. This is particularly important for melons that have a porous rind, such as cantaloupe, which can harbor salmonella — no, thanks. You definitely don't want that to get into the fruit, and you don't want it on your hands, which is all the more reason for washing.

2. **Lay the cantaloupe on a cutting board.**

3. **Cut the cantaloupe in half using a long knife.**

4. **Use a tablespoon or a larger spoon to scoop the seeds out of each half. Also scoop out the mush that was holding the seeds in place.**

5. **Slice the melon into slivers/wedges.**

The skinny on watermelon seeds

It's hard to imagine a watermelon without the seeds, even though there are those suspicious seedless watermelons. In a regular watermelon, ever notice that there are black seeds and white seeds? What's the difference, besides color and size? Why are they different?

It's all about age. Watermelon seeds start off white and small, and then grow and become black, tan, reddish, or spotted (but in most watermelon, the seeds are plain black). By the time a watermelon is ripe, almost all the seeds have matured into black seeds. However, about 5 percent are immature and are still small and white. There's nothing wrong with them, though — those white seeds require less chewing and are easier to eat than the black seeds. Any watermelon seed is edible.

Don't believe what your uncle used to tell you about how if you eat a watermelon seed you'll grow a watermelon in your belly. Nope. In fact, the seeds are very nutritious and high in protein. Just chew carefully.

Now what's with those seedless watermelons we mentioned? Those seeds aren't quite seeds. See, they're sterile. Crack inside them, and you'll see they're empty.

You can stop there, or cut the rind away from the flesh. You can then cut the melon into cubes or do something crazy like make it into spears or cut it out with cookie cutters. But really, there's nothing wrong with simple cubes. Or scoop with a melon baller!

Oatmeal

Oatmeal is a nice neutral food. Some people would say it's bland. But it doesn't have to be! Oatmeal takes on flavor really well, so throw in a little brown sugar, a dash of salt, and you just might like that oatmeal. These are also nice additions to oatmeal:

- ✔ Dried fruit
- ✔ Fresh fruit
- ✔ Milk
- ✔ Nuts
- ✔ Seeds

Oatmeal is gentle, and for that reason, it's especially good for people who have acid reflux, but it's also an overall healthy food. Oats are high in fiber, but not the kind of fiber that causes gas, so this is a low-bloat food. Oats are high in magnesium and anti-inflammatory.

Inflammation is the root of a staggering amount of illnesses — from cancer to heart disease — so any time you find a food that lowers inflammation, it's a food to pay attention to.

You don't have to eat oatmeal to enjoy oats. Instead, try muesli — there's a nice recipe for muesli in Chapter 9.

Tofu

Again, neutrality is the theme. Tofu is a low-acid food. Very low. Plus, it's a fantastic source of protein. So, instead of getting your protein only through fatty sources such as red meat, try mixing things up by bringing tofu into your diet.

In Asia, tofu is extremely popular, but in the United States, tofu has a bad reputation with a lot of people. They're put off by the name, by how white and square it is, and by how bland tofu is on its own.

Think of tofu like a potato — it's tasteless alone, but flavor it up and cook it properly and you have a nice little flavor vessel.

So, what is tofu? It's made of soybeans. The soybeans are cooked and fermented and poured into a rectangle mold. That's why the hunk of it you get in that little plastic container is so very geometric. Tofu can be flavored and prepared in myriad ways, so even if you've had it a few times and didn't like it, try it again in a different dish. You may find that you love it!

Some people like tofu raw, but that's definitely not the most popular way to have it. Tofu is very good marinated and either sautéed, baked, grilled, or roasted. It's good fried, too, but steer away from frying if you have acid reflux.

Rice

There are so many types of rice, and not one — not one! — is an acid reflux trigger. It's the way that people flavor and cook rice that can make it bad for reflux. Fried rice, for instance, can trigger acid reflux (because it's fried), and Spanish rice can as well (because it has a lot of tomato and can also have onions, chili, and garlic).

There are several rice recipes in this book. If you get tired of one type of rice, you can substitute it for another. All rice options are good, but every rice is better than white rice. White rice is much more processed than brown rice, for example. Does that mean white rice is bad for you? No. It's just not nearly as high in fiber or nutrients as its less-processed counterparts such as wild rice.

Avocado

Ahhh, fat. And the healthy kind! Yes! There are lots of reasons to love avocados. Chief among them: They have monounsaturated fat (a good fat) that can reduce bad cholesterol levels.

Avocado is bland on its own, but it comes alive with just a bit of salt. And of course, it's delicious when made into guacamole. Guacamole often contains garlic, jalapeños, lime, and onion, though, so include less guacamole in your diet, or avoid it completely. That doesn't have to change your Mexican food much, though — simply smash the avocado and combine with salt and it will still be wonderful with those tortilla chips, in burritos, or on tacos.

Non-hydrogenated products

Non-hydrogenated products have fat that stays solid at room temperature. So, to eliminate these products from your diet, you need to avoid butter, lard, vegetable shortening, frosting, and the many baked foods that contain them. The most common way to consume hydrogenated fats is in baked goods. Simply replace these foods with non-hydrogenated products (see the nutritious oils in the next section) or eat extremely small quantities.

Hydrogenation is a process that uses a stabilizer to turn oil into a solid fat. The high-fat content of these foods and the hydrogenation process itself make them difficult to digest.

Can you still eat a little butter on your toast though? Absolutely. Just keep the amounts small. As for lard or vegetable shortening, substitute oil instead. Regarding frosting, how much frosting does any of us need anyway? Okay, maybe a little. Just a little. Again, keep those portions small.

Nutritious oils

Instead of consuming hydrogenated products, consume nutritious oils instead. Every liquid oil is healthier than fats that are solid at room temperature, so cut out that vegetable shortening and reach for the corn oil or vegetable oil instead. Nut and seed oils are also good choices, and olive oil is the best.

Olive oil is healthy and also helps us feel satisfied, but without that distended yucky feeling of other fats, according to studies. One study, a 2013 study at Technische Universität München (TUM), a German university, showed that test subjects in a three-month trial felt more satisfied after consuming food with olive oil than food with lard, butter, or rapeseed oil. And miracle of miracles, no study participant increased in body fat or weight even after increasing olive oil consumption.

All oil is high in fat, so even nutritious oils should be consumed in moderation.

Licorice root

The first thing most of us think of when we think of licorice is the candy form. The quintessential flavor of real licorice comes from the oil in the woody part of the licorice plant. However, many "licorice" products are actually flavored with anise oil, which tastes similar to licorice (and similar to fennel, coincidentally).

The licorice that's best for acid reflux is licorice the plant. The plant is used to flavor foods, and the root is used to make medicine. Licorice root can treat digestive disorders such as heartburn, stomach inflammation, constipation, and ulcers. It's also used in throat lozenges and teas to soothe the throat. Licorice root not only helps prevent acid reflux, but also helps ease symptoms if acid reflux does occur.

How does licorice work? The chemicals in it are thought to increase the chemicals in our own bodies that decrease swelling, thin mucus, and soothe coughs.

To make a licorice tea, follow these steps:

1. **Buy a licorice root (available at some natural grocery stores).**

2. **Cut the licorice root into roughly ½-x-½-inch chunks and lay them between two layers of wax paper.**

3. **Firmly tap the licorice root with a meat cleaver or roll over it firmly with a rolling pin until the pieces are smaller and a little mushy.**

   This is not a fine science, so don't stress about the details.

4. **Put these pieces into a mortar and grind until smooth.**

5. **For each cup of tea you'd like to make, put ½ teaspoon of the mixture into a square of cheesecloth and tie it into a bundle, or use a mesh tea steeper.**

6. **Add 1 cup of water to a tea kettle for each cup of tea you'd like to make.**

7. **Bring the water to a boil. Remove from the burner.**

8. **Add the cheesecloth bundles, or the tea steeper, to the water.**

9. **Allow the tea to steep for about 8 minutes.**

10. **Pour the tea and sweeten as desired.**

Licorice isn't for everyone, but if you like black jelly beans, you'll probably like anything with licorice flavoring, including this soothing tea.

Parsley

Parsley is an herb that has been used as food and medicine for thousands of years. Parsley is used in many cultures to treat a wide variety of illnesses, from urinary tract infections to gastrointestinal illnesses such as indigestion and constipation. Parsley can also soothe the throat, which is partly why it's good for people with acid reflux.

Parsley is much more than a plate decoration. It contains oils and flavonoids that give it medicinal properties.

This leafy green is native to the Mediterranean area and was used as medicine before it was used as a food. A food, however, it is, and a healthy one at that. Parsley contains

- ✔ Calcium
- ✔ Copper
- ✔ Fiber
- ✔ Folate
- ✔ Iron
- ✔ Magnesium
- ✔ Manganese
- ✔ Phosphorus
- ✔ Potassium
- ✔ Vitamin A
- ✔ Vitamin B3
- ✔ Vitamin B12
- ✔ Vitamin C
- ✔ Vitamin K
- ✔ Zinc

Parsley is healthier fresh than dried. Flat-leaf parsley and its bushier "curled parsley" counterpart (the leaves of curled parsley are thicker, darker, and scrunched up) are equally healthy.

Very few dishes make parsley a focal point besides the Middle Eastern dish tabbouleh (which combines it with trigger foods such as garlic, lemon, mint, onions, and tomatoes). However, there are other ways to enjoy parsley, such as by adding a heavy garnish of it to almost any dish, throwing it in soups and salads, or adding it to pesto (go easy on the garlic if you're eating pesto and have acid reflux).

Planning menus for the week ahead

Any diet is easier if you're organized, so make a food plan. Planning will be especially important in the beginning of the diet, at least for the first week. See what recipes you like the most in the first week, and then set up a meal plan for the rest of the month, highlighting those favorite recipes.

Why do you only need a food plan for the first few weeks or months? Because your choices will become second nature after that. In the meantime, go in armed with a mission.

- ✔ **Start with the beginning of your work or school week.** Assuming you have a standard Monday-through-Friday work or school week, make your food plan start on Sunday or Monday.

- ✔ **Write down the recipes you're going to make for each day in that next week.** Sometimes, you won't need a recipe. For instance, maybe for breakfast you're going to keep having your same old oatmeal, if that's what you like and if you're sure it's not worsening your reflux. If it ain't broke, keep eating it.

- ✔ **Do your shopping the day before you start, or earlier.** Make sure you have food for three meals a day and snacks for the next week. Yes, this diet is more about eliminating and reducing foods than it is about adding them, but you'll be able to stick to it better if you have lots of foods that work for you on hand.

Do you need to plot your every snack? No. And if you plan to make a certain meal for dinner on Tuesday, do you need to stick to that plan, come hell or high water? No. You can switch it with the meal you had planned for Friday, or Wednesday, or whatever floats your boat. Flexibility is key!

Cooking with Acid Reflux in Mind

You may not need to change your cooking habits much to accommodate your reflux. Yay!

The main cooking point to keep in mind is that fried foods exacerbate acid reflux. So, here's an easy fix: Stop frying foods, or at least do it rarely. And when you do fry, eat a very small portion.

Almost anything that can be fried can be baked, roasted, or sautéed instead. Often, the most delicious alternative to frying is sautéing.

It's easy. Let's say you love sliced potatoes and you're used to deep-fat frying them. Well, no matter how tasty those fried taters may turn out, you don't need acidic fiery memories of them at midnight when you're trying to sleep, right? Right. So, try sautéing them instead. Here's how:

1. **Turn a burner onto medium heat.**

2. **Put a frying pan or sauté pan on the burner and let the pan heat up for a minute or two.**

Understanding pH balance

This chapter mentions "low-acid foods" several times. What exactly does low-acid mean? Understanding the pH balance is part of getting started on the reflux diet.

The categorization of low acid versus high acid has to do with where a food falls on the pH scale. Remember those TV commercials that advertised shampoos with the "right pH balance"? Well, finding foods with the right pH balance is more important than finding pH-balanced shampoo, if you're prone to acid reflux.

The pH scale is used to measure acidity and alkalinity, and everything in between. Keep in mind that the opposite of acid isn't "the absence of acid." The opposite of complete acid is complete alkalinity. That's why the pH scale is a little more confusing than most scales. A pH of 0 is totally acidic, while a pH of 14 is completely alkaline. A pH of 7 is neutral.

Most water is close to pH 7 (neutral), whereas vinegar is pH 2.9 and lemon juice is pH 2.7. The normal level of stomach acid has a pH ranging from 1.5 to 3.5, but usually around 2. The hydrochloric acid that makes up stomach acid is some pretty impressive stuff. Fortunately, your stomach lining secretes mucous to coat the interior and protect itself against being burned or ulcerated.

You know about many foods that are acidic (citrus, tomatoes, and so on), but there are also acidic additives to be on the lookout for. Avoid these additives if you want to avoid reflux:

✔ Ascorbic acid

✔ Citric acid

✔ Phosphoric acid

✔ Anything labeled "Vitamin C added"

You may hear people say that they're on an alkaline diet. That means they're eating foods that are as close to neutral on the pH scale as possible. That means eating lots of fruits (except citrus) and vegetables, and avoiding foods that are acidic or that cause a lot of acid, such as red meat. Alkaline diets are similar to the acid reflux diet. The foods that you're supposed to eat on an alkaline diet are good for you (lean meats, lots of water, no soda) and are good for avoiding reflux as well.

Are you curious about the acid levels in your esophagus? There's a way to test them. It's called the 48-hour Bravo esophageal pH test. We cover this procedure briefly in Chapter 2. The test measures and records the pH in your esophagus and can determine whether you have gastroesophageal reflux disease (GERD). It measures how often stomach contents reflux into the lower esophagus and how much acid the reflux contains.

Remember: You don't have to do this test to find out whether you have acid reflux. If you have acid reflux, you know you have acid reflux. However, it wouldn't hurt to get a number on just how bad yours is. Such information can be valuable in getting you started on the acid reflux diet.

3. **Pour a tablespoon or two of oil into the pan, depending on how many potato slices you're cooking.**

   Olive oil is a particularly good choice because it's a healthier fat than vegetable oil. Plus, olive oil is also far healthier than any fat that stays solid at room temperature, such as butter, lard, or Crisco.

4. **Allow the oil to get hot.**

   This will only take a minute or two. If you want to season the oil, go for it — try a little salt and pepper and/or herbs (fresh or dried).

   Swirl the pan around so the oil distributes evenly. When there's a little smoke coming off the oil or when the pepper starts to cook, you know the oil is hot enough for the potatoes.

5. **Put the potatoes into the pan. Cover with a lid.**

6. **Cook until the potatoes are soft and one side is golden brown, and then flip them.**

7. **Keep the lid off and cook until both sides are golden brown.**

Chapter 7

That Thing You Do: Embracing Lifestyle Changes

*W*hen acid reflux has you down, take comfort in this: You have the power to make some key lifestyle changes that can keep acid reflux at bay! And the good news is, all these changes will have positive effects in the rest of your life, too. You can feel better and look better, all while slaying the acid reflux dragon. In this chapter, we show you how.

If you and change aren't best friends, and you're resisting altering your lifestyle in any way, keep in mind this old adage: "If you keep doing what you're doing, you're going to keep getting what you've got." If you want to change your situation (a burning throat), you'll probably have to change your lifestyle a bit.

Start with one change at a time, and stick with it until it's old hat. Then add another change to the mix, and see how you feel. If you're still experiencing symptoms of acid reflux, make another change, and so on. Before you know it, you'll have made some pretty significant changes to your lifestyle.

Paying Attention to How Much You Eat and When You Eat It

When it comes to acid reflux, one of the first areas to look at is your diet — not just what you're eating, but how much and when. Every aspect of your diet can affect the severity of your symptoms. Changing your eating habits can be a relatively simple and inexpensive way to reduce the inflammation and pain caused by reflux.

Reducing the amount you eat at one sitting

The specific foods that trigger acid reflux differ from person to person, but the impact of a giant meal does not. The human digestive system doesn't do well when we jam it with too much food. The most common time people suffer from reflux symptoms is right after a hefty meal. A simple calorie- and fat-laden trip to your favorite fast-food restaurant for a deluxe bacon cheeseburger, super-sized fries, and a milkshake can lead to hours of searing discomfort.

When you eat, your stomach expands to make room for the food. The more you eat, the more your stomach has to expand. This expansion increases the amount of pressure on your *lower esophageal sphincter* (LES), the muscle responsible for keeping stomach acid from escaping into your esophagus.

A good rule of thumb is to eat a meal the size of your cupped hands or smaller. That doesn't sound like much, right? Well, the stomach isn't very big, and it's not good to stretch it out too far. *Remember:* The crucial factor here is not *what* you're eating, but how much. When consumed in large quantities, even reflux-friendly foods can trigger the burn.

Not overloading the stomach is one of the reasons doctors and nutritionists recommend eating five or six small meals a day instead of the traditional three meals a day you grew up on. An added bonus: Spacing your meals evenly throughout the day will help keep your blood sugar steady, which will make you feel less hungry, and all that will make you less likely to binge. Small meals mean less stress on the stomach and less stress on the LES (say that five times fast) and, therefore, less heartburn.

Depending on your schedule, finding the time to eat several small meals throughout the day can be difficult. This is where planning ahead becomes critical. Start with the foundation of a good breakfast. You can still have lunch and dinner at regular times, but eat less than usual. In between those meals, snack on healthy, reflux-friendly foods — three snacks a day will do the trick.

If you eat most of your meals away from home, you may have noticed that many restaurants serve meals that are significantly larger than what dietitians and nutritionists recommend. This is one of the few times in life when it's okay to disregard what your parents taught you: You don't have to clear your plate. Take the rest home with you in a doggie bag!

Timing your meals with acid reflux in mind

When you eat can be just as important as how much you eat. Eating a meal right before lying down on the couch or going to bed can quickly turn a delicious meal into a catalyst for suffering.

Lying down right after a meal makes stomach emptying slower and increases the odds that you'll experience reflux symptoms. Always allow at least two hours for your food to leave your stomach before you lie down. This means avoiding the temptation of late-night snacks. Standing up and moving around gently for about 30 minutes after a meal can also reduce your chances of experiencing reflux symptoms.

A reflux diary can be a valuable tool. An honest and detailed journal can help you and your doctor assess the causes and severity of your reflux. Be sure to write down

- ✔ When and what you eat
- ✔ When and what exercises you do
- ✔ When and what medications and supplements you take
- ✔ When you experience pain or other reflux symptoms
- ✔ A description of the pain or symptoms
- ✔ Anything you do that reduces those symptoms

Suck it up: Laying off the straws

It's not just what you drink that can affect your reflux, but also how you drink it. The simple act of drinking from a straw can inflame your throat. As strange as it may seem, choosing to drink straight from a cup instead of a straw can have an impact. Drinking out of a straw causes a siphon like effect, pulling gastric contents up your esophagus. Think of the tube you use to siphon gas from a car gas tank — same deal.

Losing Weight

Anyone of any size can suffer from acid reflux — if you have a stomach and an esophagus, you're fair game. It doesn't matter if you're at a healthy weight or obese — you can still experience that troublesome burn. However, excess weight *does* increase your chances of developing acid reflux, and if you already have acid reflux, the state of being overweight can make it worse.

Recent research has shown just how much impact body weight can have. Gaining even a few extra pounds can be the catalyst for heartburn. An increase of 10 to 20 pounds makes you *three times* more likely to experience reflux symptoms. The good news is that shedding just a few excess pounds can reduce or even eliminate reflux from your life.

While the link between excess weight and acid reflux has been proven, researchers have yet to identify the precise reason weight has such an impact. The most commonly accepted explanation is that excess weight increases the pressure on the abdominal cavity, and this extra pressure can result in the stomach forcing acid into the esophagus.

For some people, shedding just a few pounds may be the key to eliminating acid reflux. This is welcome information for anyone who can't imagine a life without hot sauce. Plus, losing weight has other benefits outside of reducing or eliminating your acid reflux. Shedding excess pounds also reduces your risk for other significant health issues, such as heart disease and diabetes. And you'll never get tired of looking and feeling better and hearing your friends and family talk about how great you look!

Daily physical exercise is one way you can cut weight and maintain or improve overall health. Aim for about 30 minutes of physical activity every day. You don't have to sign up for an expensive gym membership or book time with a personal trainer. A good old-fashioned walk or leisurely bike ride can help you drop a few pounds and improve your overall health.

In addition to physical activity, another important key to losing weight is cutting calories. Cutting calories doesn't mean you have to starve or eat tasteless food or follow the latest trendy diet. Studies have shown that reducing your daily caloric intake is more important than eliminating fat, carbs, or protein from your diet — besides, you need fat, carbs, and protein! Aim for cutting between 500 to 1,000 calories per day and a modest weight loss target of 1 to 2 pounds a week. You may lose more weight with more severe diets, but you're also significantly more likely to gain that weight back as soon as you get off the diet, and who knows what strange side effects you'll get from a diet of, say, all grapefruit?

Small changes, big results

Meet Joe, an Arizona resident. Last year, Joe started suffering severe bouts of reflux-induced heartburn. It was bad enough that he was losing sleep. A trip to the doctor confirmed his acid reflux and led to a prescription for Prilosec. On top of the medicine, Joe's doctor told him to lose weight, cut his caffeine intake, and eliminate spicy foods from his life. Coffee and spicy food just happened to be two of Joe's favorite things.

Joe cut his calories so drastically (to about 1,000 calories a day) that he was practically starving. Between that and eliminating coffee and spicy foods from his life, he wasn't happy.

A few weeks later, he was still struggling to adjust to these changes. Although his reflux was no longer causing him sleepless nights, he felt deprived and was irritated about being told what to eat and drink. His doctor shared some recent studies linking weight and acid reflux, and suggested that it may be a better option to cut calories less dramatically, and to eat less of his favorite foods instead of eliminating them completely.

Joe increased his daily caloric intake to around 1,700, and had a little bit of coffee and small, infrequent servings of spicy foods. Over the next three weeks, he lost 8 pounds and said he was feeling better every week. After four months, he had lost 23 pounds and hadn't experienced acid reflux symptoms in more than a month!

Joe was able to stop taking his reflux medication, and now he happily enjoys a small cup of joe (no pun intended) and the occasional visit to his favorite Thai restaurant.

Quitting Smoking

Just like losing weight, quitting smoking is something every doctor recommends. Doctors make those recommendations for overall health purposes, but does quitting smoking impact something as specific as acid reflux? The answer is yes! In fact, it isn't just the act of smoking that has a link to reflux, but tobacco itself.

Any form of tobacco — from cigarettes to cigars, pipes, chew, or snuff — can trigger acid reflux. So, cutting back (and hopefully quitting tobacco completely) can not only reduce the intensity of your symptoms, but also potentially eliminate reflux from your life altogether.

What exactly is it about smoking and tobacco that can cause acid reflux and increase its severity?

- ✔ **Increased acid production:** Nicotine has been shown to increase stomach acid production. More stomach acid means a higher chance that some of that acid may be pushed out of the stomach and into the esophagus.

✔ **Reduced pressure of the LES:** Again, nicotine is the primary culprit, because it reduces pressure in the LES. When the LES is too lax, it allows stomach acid to creep up into your throat. No bueno.

✔ **Irritated esophagus:** Tobacco smoke has been shown to irritate and inflame the esophageal lining, causing and intensifying that all-too-familiar burning sensation.

✔ **Reduced saliva production:** Saliva is actually good for reducing acid reflux: The more saliva, the less acid reflux. Saliva contains an acid neutralizer called bicarbonate, which can help minimize damage to your esophagus. Tobacco slows saliva production, which takes away some of your protection.

Most research examining tobacco's impact on acid reflux has revolved around smoking, but nicotine, which is present in all forms of tobacco, can also increase reflux and amplify its symptoms. Unfortunately, this means that switching to a nicotine patch or gum won't necessarily reduce your reflux symptoms. This move will, however, stop the damage that smoke does to your esophagus and decrease your risk for lung disease, heart disease, and cancer. So, don't hesitate to switch over to patches or gum, especially if it's the first step on your journey to quitting tobacco all together.

Tobacco may also increase the amount of damage acid reflux does to your esophagus. Not only are you more likely to suffer long-term effects, such as chronic inflammation or even esophageal cancer, but your body will take longer to heal than it would take somebody who doesn't smoke.

Even a slight reduction in the amount you smoke can have a positive impact on your reflux symptoms. More exciting is that you could begin to notice a difference just a few days after cutting back or stopping.

It's important to note that quitting smoking is not guaranteed to eliminate reflux. Some physicians maintain that smoking only has a moderate impact. But even if quitting smoking doesn't totally cure your acid reflux, there are enough medical benefits to make this change worth the effort.

Managing Stress

Have you ever noticed that your acid reflux seems to kick in at the most inconvenient times? It could be just before a big meeting or when you're trying to get a good night's sleep before a big speech. Well, it's not a coincidence: Stress can trigger acid reflux.

Stress doesn't just affect your mind — it actually causes physiological changes in your body. Because your body doesn't differentiate between external and internal threats, it reacts the same way to mental stress as it would if you were being chased by a pack of rabid dogs. The blood shunts to your legs — great for running like heck — and away from the gastrointestinal tract. That adrenaline rush can be helpful in small doses, but not when it's common and over a long period of time. Prolonged stress can affect every aspect of your life, including acid reflux.

Stress can have many different causes, and what stresses you out may not have any effect on anyone else you know. Stress can be a result of almost anything from health issues to emotional problems, relationship issues, major life changes, business issues, or even just your environment. Stress doesn't necessarily come from something negative either. Positive changes in your life — such as getting married, starting a new job, getting a promotion, or becoming a parent — can be almost as stressful as dealing with a family member's death. With so many potential causes, the first thing you need to do to address your stress is to find out what in particular stresses *you.*

Several studies have examined the kinds of stressors that most often lead to bouts of reflux. Interestingly, the most common causes of stress-related heartburn are different for men and women. Women tend to report higher incidences of heartburn due to relationship stressors, whereas men tend to link their heartburn to hectic workdays and business travel.

Regardless of the root cause, stress can create the perfect storm of anxiety and acid reflux. Research shows that prolonged stress over a six-month period leads to a significant increase in acid reflux symptoms over the following four months.

Stress may not actually increase the production of stomach acid, a common cause of acid reflux, but it does make you more sensitive to smaller amounts of acid in the esophagus. This means that your reflux may not actually be getting worse, but it will feel like it is.

You feel the effects of reflux when you're stressed because stress triggers chemical changes in the brain that increase the sensitivity of pain receptors. This means you'll feel even a tiny amount of stomach acid in your esophagus. Stress also affects the production of *prostaglandin,* a lipid compound that helps protect your stomach from being damaged by acid. Less prostaglandin means more discomfort.

Stress reduction techniques can reduce your acid reflux symptoms. Although there are a wide variety of stress reduction methods, finding the one that works best for you is essential. Some of the most common ways to reduce stress include

✔ Working out

✔ Practicing yoga, tai chi, or meditation

✔ Listening to music

✔ Going on vacation

✔ Getting a massage

✔ Doing anything creative, such as painting or drawing

✔ Talking with a friend

✔ Spending time with people who calm you down

✔ De-cluttering your environment

✔ Taking on fewer tasks

✔ Going for slow walks

✔ Getting more sleep

✔ Having sex

If these approaches don't do the trick, you may want to consider visiting a cognitive behavioral therapist. A good therapist can help you restructure negative thinking in an effort to reduce stress.

Keeping a journal can help you identify key stressors and help you evaluate the effectiveness of your coping strategies. Be sure to include what was going on at the time you noticed your stress begin to appear, as well as what you did to cope with it and whether you felt it reduced your stress level. Scoring your stress level from 1 to 10 will help you standardize your results. Keep in mind that some coping methods, such as drinking alcohol, smoking, or overeating, may make you feel better in the short term, but they'll end up doing more harm than good in the long term.

Figuring out what specific stressors affect your reflux and which coping methods are most effective will have benefits outside of simply reducing your reflux symptoms. Stress reduction will help nearly every other part of your life. High levels of stress have been linked to

✔ Anxiety and depression

✔ Memory loss

✔ Insomnia

✔ Irritability and moodiness

✔ Physical aches

✔ High blood pressure

✔ Heart attacks

✔ Strokes

A little bit of stress can be a good thing, helping you to stay focused, alert, and energetic. But prolonged periods of heightened stress can have serious consequences for your overall health, and your esophagus.

Looking At How You Sleep: Position, Position, Position

Loss of sleep is the most common complaint from people who have heartburn. Sixty percent of Americans with chronic acid reflux report experiencing heartburn at night.

Donna, a 55-year-old woman, is a perfect example of how acid reflux can impact sleeping patterns. For the past few years, Donna has been struggling with nighttime heartburn from her acid reflux. In a typical week, she experiences reflux symptoms two or three times, usually a few hours before bedtime. Getting into bed when her symptoms flare up is not an option, unless Donna decides that having acid burn her throat and into her nose is something she wants. Lying down increases the intensity of her symptoms to the point where sleep is the last thing on her mind. No amount of antacids or medication makes a difference. To get any rest, she has to sleep upright in a reclining chair.

Donna is onto the right idea, because gravity can be one of the most effective ways to combat nighttime acid reflux. When you lie down after eating, it makes it easier for stomach acid to move up your esophagus. Slightly elevating your head and shoulders allows gravity to help keep the acid down, which often reduces heartburn.

Try raising the head of your bed by about 6 inches. Placing blocks or pillows underneath the mattress can be the most effective way to do this. This approach isn't always an option, especially if your significant other doesn't suffer from reflux, or you sleep on a water bed. If you can't elevate the head of your bed, you may want to invest in a specially designed wedge pillow (see Figure 7-1). Stacking regular pillows is an option, but make sure to create a level incline down to your hips, otherwise you put excess strain on your neck and shoulders, and squish your abdomen, raising the stomach pressure and promoting reflux.

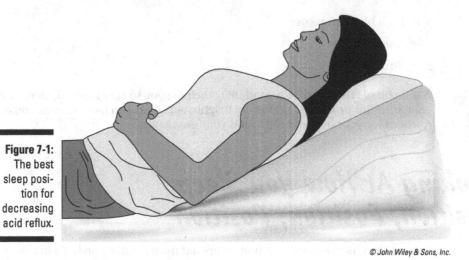

Figure 7-1:
The best sleep position for decreasing acid reflux.

You can also try sleeping on your left side. Lying on your left side aids the stomach emptying by putting the outflow of the stomach downstream, reducing the likelihood that you'll experience reflux symptoms.

Chapter 8

Staying Fit, Inside and Out

. . . .

In This Chapter

▶ Recognizing the benefits of exercise

▶ Trying relaxation techniques

▶ Joining a support group

. . . .

The main benefit of being active is that exercise helps you achieve and maintain a healthy weight. Excess weight puts too much pressure on the lower esophageal sphincter (LES), and that pressure can cause acid reflux.

People who are overweight are much more likely to suffer from acid reflux than people who are at a healthy weight. To reach or maintain a healthy weight, it's all about calories in versus calories out. Americans tend to over-complicate this issue. Yes, every now and then someone has a condition (such as a thyroid problem) that makes it especially difficult to lose weight, but the vast majority of people who don't have such conditions can lose weight. How? Through this process: Burn more calories than you consume.

It really is that simple. Now, simple doesn't mean easy. We all know that losing weight is tough. But again, tough doesn't mean complicated. Even if you eat unhealthy foods, if you're only eating, say, 1,100 calories a day, you'll lose weight. You could go on an all-Twizzlers diet and lose weight, but you won't be healthy. That's why it's much smarter to eat healthy foods *and* reduce your calorie count. One more tenet of this trifecta? Exercise.

Getting Physical

Everyone knows that exercise is good. You can maintain a healthy weight or even lose weight without exercise, but you won't be as healthy. Exercise gives you more energy, helps you live longer, and often makes you look healthier, not just because of a healthy weight, but because sweating is good for the skin and gives the skin a nice glow.

Here are some more ways that exercise can improve your life

✔ **Exercise helps prevent a long list of things you don't want.** The list includes heart disease, high blood pressure, arthritis, diabetes, some forms of cancer, stroke, and depression.

✔ **Exercise can make you happier.** Can't we all use all the emotional boosts we can get? Exercise has been proven to put people in a better mood. Now, you may hate exercising while you're doing it, but afterward, chances are, you'll feel pretty darned good, or at least better.

How does this work? Exercise evokes chemicals in the brain that just plain make you more relaxed and happier. Getting this chemical boost or "natural high" doesn't require running a marathon. Even a 20-minute walk will do the trick.

Need an emotional lift? Or need to blow off some steam after a stressful day? A workout at the gym or a brisk 30-minute walk can help. Physical activity stimulates various brain chemicals that may leave you feeling happier and more relaxed. You may also feel better about your appearance and yourself when you exercise regularly, which can boost your confidence and improve your self-esteem.

✔ **Exercise helps you sleep better.** Exercise can help you fall asleep, stay asleep, and sleep more deeply. There can be a little catch, though: For some people, exercising too close to bedtime can keep them wired and then they have a hard time falling asleep. Other people, however, like to exercise close to bedtime. So, try both and see which works for you.

✔ **Exercise can ramp up your sex life.** Some people feel too tired, winded, or unattractive to get "in the mood." Exercise, however, can turn this around by providing energy, improving longevity, and helping a person feel more confident and attractive. Studies have shown that regular exercise increases arousal for women. And men who exercise regularly are less likely to have erectile dysfunction.

For people with bad acid reflux, their sex lives may already be impaired. Who feels sexy when they're uncomfortable, grouchy, not sleeping well, and have acid burning up their esophagus? Not so many of us. Because exercise can reduce acid reflux by maintaining a healthy weight, and exercise helps people feel more aroused and more desirable, it's clearly a win-win for the bedroom.

✔ **Exercise can be fun!** All right, you may be rolling your eyes, and maybe rolling your eyes is all the exercise you want to do. Ever. Fair enough. However, challenge yourself to find some form of exercise that you actually like. How about a fast walk? Okay, even a slow walk. Leg lifts on the couch when you're watching television? Yoga? Dancing? Going to the gym? Tennis? Aerobics on a DVD in the privacy of your living room?

Most people can go for a walk, so at least try that. Getting outside or in a different environment can help change your perspective and can be an excuse to meet new people, or to strengthen friendships by exercising with someone else. And if you can't go for a walk, don't let that stop you from exercising — maybe you can swim or do chair aerobics!

If you're new to exercise, take it easy in the beginning. If you decide to hit the gym, don't make that first session a two-hour grueling ordeal. Start off nice and slow. Starting a yoga class? Take a beginner's class, not something advanced.

How often to exercise and how much are very individual factors. Take into consideration your current fitness level. If you have no clue what level of exercise you should take up, consult your doctor or a sports therapist. Consider consulting a trainer in the beginning to make certain you have proper form.

Yes, exercise is a part of overall health and can reduce acid reflux, but there's a catch. Some people report that certain types of exercise make their heartburn worse. Oh no! Forms of exercise that kick up the acid for some people include running, jumping rope, aerobics, abdominal exercises (such as sit-ups), high-activity dance (think Zumba, not the waltz), anything that puts you upside down (such as a headstand in yoga), and anything that reverses the flow of gravity.

You don't have to be fully upside down for the flow of gravity to be reversed. For instance, just touching your toes reverses the flow of gravity.

Fortunately, most forms of exercise either won't bother your reflux or can be modified so that they're more gentle. The more boisterous, jumpy, and jerky a form of exercise is, the more likely it is to cause acid reflux. Some great forms of exercise that most people with reflux find enjoyable include walking, swimming, and bike riding.

The likelihood of exercise triggering reflux is higher if someone has a weak or relaxed LES. This weak or relaxed state is often the case in people who have suffered from acid reflux for a long period of time. Enough acid, enough damage, and that LES pays the price.

The same foods that make heartburn bad also make exercise more painful. So, if that glass of orange juice in the morning already bothers you an hour later, it's going to bother you double if you go for a jog right after you drink it. This doesn't mean you should avoid exercise. It just means you should avoid trigger foods, especially when you're going to exercise, and you should modify or avoid boisterous, jumpy, jerky, or upside-down exercise.

Try these exercise tips to avoid or reduce exercise-induced acid reflux:

✔ **Avoid eating for at least two hours before you exercise, and make sure to avoid your trigger foods.** If salsa bothers you and you're going to splurge and go to a salsa festival, don't jog when you get home.

✔ **Now this may sound contradictory to the previous tip, but some people do better exercising when they have a little snack in their system.** Again, the snack should not contain your trigger foods. And the keyword is *snack,* not meal. If you choose a safe form of exercise, and you avoid eating for a couple hours before exercising, and you *still* feel that the physical activity gave you reflux, try eating a snack an hour before you exercise. The snack should be mild — for example, half of a banana or a little yogurt may do the trick.

✔ **An hour before you exercise, take an antacid.** Granted, antacids are meant for symptom relief, not for prevention, but there is some evidence that antacids can work as preventive measures. Don't make this a routine, however. Using an antacid should be looked at as a crutch as you're beginning your new diet and exercise regime. When you eliminate trigger foods, increase calming foods, and find the exercise types that work for you, your body very well may regulate and you may not need that antacid.

For many people, heartburn feels like a heart attack, and a heart attack can feel just like reflux — so don't blow it off! If your pain or discomfort is anything even *slightly* different from or more serious than your usual heartburn pain or discomfort, call 911, especially if you're overweight, you've had a heart attack, or you're over 40. Chest pain should not be taken lightly.

Focusing Inward

Physical activity is essential for health, but health isn't just about breaking a sweat. It's also about focusing inward — finding ways to calm your mind and reduce stress. You can use meditation, journaling, and support groups to address your acid reflux. No sweat required.

Meditation and other relaxation techniques

How does relaxation help with acid reflux? The link isn't iron clad. However, relaxation does promote overall health, and if you improve your overall health your acid reflux may decrease.

Here are some basic tips for relaxation:

✔ **Turn off the television when you're trying to sleep.** Studies are clear that the brain does not "sleep" as well when the television is on, even if it's on mute.

✔ **Keep your bedroom as dark as possible when you're sleeping.**

✔ **Exercise.** As mentioned, exercise helps people feel more relaxed.

✔ **If you're feeling upset, take a break from the situation.** Even if it's a high-pressure board meeting, maybe you can get away with a quick trip to the restroom. Breathe deeply, close your eyes, and remind yourself that whatever is happening will probably improve. Examine whether you're making a mountain out of a mole hill and feeling unnecessary stress.

✔ **Keep your environment as relaxing as possible.** Do you like soothing colors? Soothing music? Soothing foods? Do certain people make you feel stressed out? Avoid those people! Seek out what makes you feel peaceful.

You can also practice relaxation techniques. Deep breathing is about as simple as it gets. Try this: Stop for a moment. Close your eyes. Inhale deeply and slowly, engaging your stomach as though you're pulling the air up from your stomach, instead of just engaging your chest. Pause. Release. Take another deep, slow breath. Pause. Release. Take another deep, slow breath. Pause. Release. To see whether you're doing this correctly, place a hand on your belly and a hand on your chest. Your belly should move when you take a deep breath, but your chest and shoulders should not.

You know it's working when you feel calmer. If you don't feel calmer yet, breathe deeper, slower, and for longer. If you still can't calm down, consider consulting medical help.

If you're interested in taking it another step, you can practice meditation. We don't have room to go into detail on meditation in this book, but check out *Meditation For Dummies,* 3rd Edition, by Stephan Bodian (Wiley). It comes with a CD of guided meditations.

There's not a direct correlation (yet, anyway) between high stress and frequent reflux, but again, if you improve your overall health, you're less likely to have acid reflux. So, de-stress. But don't stress about it.

Food journaling

At its most basic form, a *food journal* is a log of everything you eat. Keeping a food journal is most helpful if you're an emotional, distracted, or unaware eater. By writing about what you eat, you're likely to see patterns. For example, do you consume most of your sweets around 2 p.m.? What's happening around that time to make you want sweets? Is that when you have a deadline or daily meeting that stresses you out? You don't have to write a novel or a diary entry to see these patterns. For instance, just a few quick notes about what you ate and when, every meal, every snack, for a few weeks, can tell you a lot. If you have time, jot down how you're feeling when you eat, too. That way, you can track how your emotions affect your eating.

Support groups

For some people, food and exercise are private matters. For others, having support makes it all easier.

If you're not getting the support you need at home, hit up the Internet and look for an eating or exercise support group near you. There may even be support groups for folks sharing your same stressors, like groups for folks suffering from angst-laden bosses or troublesome teens. You just may come away with some new friends, healthy recipes, and an exercise buddy!

There are also online communities for people with acid reflux. These groups can provide information and support.

Part III
Symptom-Soothing Recipes

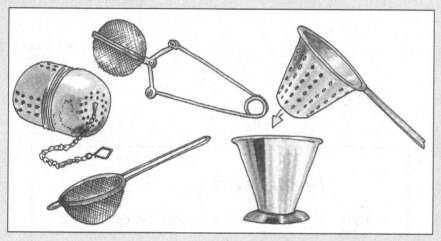

Illustration by Elizabeth Kurtzman

Find reflux-friendly snacks in a free article at www.dummies.com/extras/
acidrefluxdiet.

In this part . . .

- ✔ Find breakfast, lunch, and dinner recipes to keep your reflux at bay.
- ✔ Keep your appetizers and snacks reflux friendly.
- ✔ Hydrate and refresh with easing and pleasing beverages.
- ✔ Cap off your meal with a worry-free dessert.

Chapter 9

Beginning with Breakfast

In This Chapter

▶ Starting your day with eggs

▶ Baking your breakfast

▶ Going for grains

▶ Keeping it light with fruits and vegetables

*Y*ou know what your mom always said: "Breakfast is the most important meal of the day." Okay, maybe only June Cleaver said that. Maybe your mom skipped breakfast and didn't mind that you did, too. Either way, breakfast is important.

It gives you energy to start the day and is linked to improved health and better weight control. Studies show that people who eat breakfast regularly tend to weigh less than people who regularly skip breakfast. Morning calories improve concentration, and people who consume breakfast regularly have more strength and endurance and lower cholesterol.

You can find a ton of unhealthy choices (donuts, bacon), but breakfast also affords healthy choices, and you'll see many such choices in this chapter. Not only are these recipes healthy overall, but they're finely tuned for people who are trying to prevent acid reflux.

Eggceptional Breakfasts

Eggs got a bad rep in the 1990s, but they're actually a healthy source of protein. Sure, they have quite a bit of fat, but it's a healthy type of fat. Just limit yourself to one or two eggs a week, and refrain from frying them in lots of oil or butter.

If you're worried about cholesterol, you can leave a yolk or two out of a dish that's heavy on eggs, or thin down the eggs with lowfat milk or soymilk so that you're getting more food but fewer calories and less cholesterol.

Choosing the best eggs

Eggs are common in the Mediterranean diet because they're economical and readily available. Eggs are a great choice because they're a good source of protein and vitamins A, D, and B12. Although eggs can be part of a healthy diet, you have to handle them carefully because they may be contaminated with *salmonella,* a bacteria that can make you very sick.

Use the following tips to avoid problems:

✔ Open egg cartons before you buy them and avoid any that contain cracked or unclean eggs.

✔ Avoid purchasing eggs at room temperature, because eggs can spoil quickly when not refrigerated.

✔ Discard eggs after the expiration date on the package. If you have farm-fresh eggs, you can store them in the refrigerator for four to five weeks.

✔ Take a good look at your eggs when cooking. The egg white should be thick, and the yolk should sit firm and high rather than flat.

✔ Don't eat eggs raw. You don't know whether that particular egg contains salmonella, and cooking the eggs is the only way to destroy the bacteria.

Determining when eggs spoil is difficult because they don't change color or have an odor. To check whether your eggs are good, carefully place them in a bowl of cold water. If they sink, they're in good shape. If they float, they're old, and you should toss them out. The more they float, the older they are.

Farmer's Market Scramble

Prep time: 10 min • **Cook time:** 8 min • **Yield:** 4 servings

Ingredients	Directions
8 eggs	*1* In a bowl, whisk together the eggs, milk, and salt and pepper. Continue whisking until the eggs are frothy. Set aside.
2 tablespoons lowfat milk	
Salt and pepper, to taste	
4 teaspoons extra-virgin olive oil	*2* In a stainless-steel frying pan, warm the oil over medium heat.
1 small zucchini, diced	*3* Add the zucchini and cook, while stirring, until tender.
1 small red bell pepper, diced	
1 cup firmly packed arugula	*4* Add the bell pepper and stir to combine. Reduce the heat to medium-low. Add the arugula and let it wilt.
¼ cup grated Parmesan cheese	
	5 Add the egg mixture and let it cook, without stirring, until the eggs just begin to set, about 1 minute.
	6 Using a spatula, gently push the eggs around the pan, letting any uncooked egg run onto the bottom of the pan. Add the cheese.
	7 Mix the ingredients gently to combine and continue cooking until the eggs are completely set.

Per serving: Calories 219 (From Fat 140); Fat 16g (Saturated 5g); Cholesterol 377mg; Sodium 372mg; Carbohydrate 4g (Dietary Fiber 1g); Protein 15g.

Vary It! Don't like Parmesan cheese? Substitute any cheese you like. Flavorful cheeses will make the dish richer and yummier. You can also easily substitute the vegetables in this recipe. Eggplant, corn, asparagus? Throw them in!

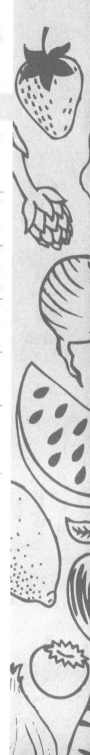

Veggie Cheese Mini Quiches

Prep time: 15 min • **Cook time:** 31–36 min • **Yield:** 6 servings

Ingredients	Directions
1 tablespoon olive oil 1 cup chopped mushrooms	*1* Preheat the oven to 350 degrees. Grease a 12-cup muffin pan with olive oil and set aside.
1 cup baby spinach leaves, chopped 4 eggs 4 egg whites	*2* In a small saucepan, heat the 1 tablespoon of olive oil over medium heat. Add the mushrooms; cook and stir for 3 minutes. Add the spinach leaves; cook for 3 minutes, or until the mushrooms are golden brown, the spinach has wilted, and the liquid has evaporated.
1/3 cup lowfat Greek or regular yogurt 1/2 teaspoon dry mustard powder 1/2 teaspoon dried thyme leaves	*3* In a medium bowl, combine the eggs, egg whites, yogurt, mustard powder, thyme, and pepper. Mix well. Stir the cheese into the egg mixture. Add the cooked vegetables to the egg and cheese mixture.
1/8 teaspoon pepper 1 cup shredded Swiss or cheddar cheese	*4* Spoon the mixture into the prepared muffin pan. Bake for 23 to 28 minutes, or until the quiches are set and light golden brown. Let them cool for 3 minutes; then run a knife around the edge of each quiche to loosen it from the pan. Remove the quiches from the pan and serve warm.

Per serving: Calories 83 (From Fat 50); Fat 6g (Saturated 2g); Cholesterol 80mg; Sodium 68mg; Carbohydrate 2g; Dietary Fiber 0g; Protein 7g.

Herb Scramble

Prep time: 10 min • **Cook time:** 5 min • **Yield:** 4 servings

Ingredients	Directions
1 bunch parsley, finely chopped	**1** Bring a medium pot of water to a boil over high heat. Add the parsley and cook for 1 minute. Drain and rinse under cold water.
8 eggs	
¼ teaspoon salt	**2** Whisk the eggs in a medium bowl. Add the parsley, salt, and pepper and whisk to combine.
¼ teaspoon pepper	
1 tablespoon extra-virgin olive oil	**3** In a large nonstick or cast-iron skillet, heat the oil over medium heat. Pour in the eggs and stir gently and constantly until the eggs form large curds and are cooked to your preference, about 2 to 3 minutes. Serve immediately.

Per serving: Calories 178 (From Fat 117); Fat 13g (Saturated 4g); Cholesterol 372mg; Sodium 296mg; Carbohydrate 2g (Dietary Fiber 1g); Protein 13g.

Tip: Have you ever been excited to use your fresh herbs only to find that they've become limp and brown, old before their time? To keep herbs fresh longer, make sure they're completely dry after you wash them. Then wrap them in plastic wrap, but not too tightly. If they're wrapped too tightly, the moisture in the leaves may promote mold. Keep the herbs in the crisper drawer in the refrigerator. Another method: Put the bottom of the stems in an inch or two of water, as though the herbs are a bouquet of flowers, and store in the fridge.

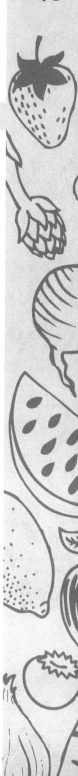

Reflux-Friendly Frittata

Prep time: 20 min • **Cook time:** 20 min • **Yield:** 6 servings

Ingredients	Directions
8 eggs	*1* Preheat the oven to 375 degrees.
¼ cup fresh basil leaves, torn	
Salt and pepper, to taste	*2* In a medium bowl, whisk together the eggs, basil, and salt and pepper. Set aside.
2 tablespoons extra-virgin olive oil	
4 small red potatoes, thinly sliced	*3* In a medium cast-iron skillet, heat the olive oil over medium heat.
6 baby portobello mushrooms, thinly sliced	*4* Add the potatoes and mushrooms to the skillet and sauté until tender, but firm, about 7 minutes.
1 cup baby spinach, torn	*5* Add the spinach to the skillet and stir it into the potato and mushroom mixture until wilted, about 1 minute.
¼ cup Parmesan cheese, for garnish	
	6 Pour the egg mixture over the vegetables and scramble for 1 minute.
	7 When the eggs have started to set around the side of the skillet, move the skillet into the oven until the eggs have set in the center, about 6 minutes.
	8 Put the oven on the broil setting. Top the eggs with the cheese and cook under the broiler for 1 or 2 minutes to melt the cheese.
	9 Serve warm, straight out of the skillet.

Per serving: Calories 236 (From Fat 107); Fat 12g (Saturated 3g); Cholesterol 251mg; Sodium 261mg; Carbohydrate 19g (Dietary Fiber 2g); Protein 12g.

Vary It! This recipe tolerates substitutions well. It also doesn't need to be measured perfectly. In short, don't stress over the ingredients. If you don't have exactly ¼ cup of basil leaves, don't worry. Less stress is good, and that calmed state may even reduce your acid reflux!

Bake It 'Til You Make It

A well-balanced carb-intensive breakfast can be a healthy choice, and with the right ingredients, it can be great for someone with acid reflux.

 Baked goods, even ones that are billed as healthy (as opposed to a donut), are an easy way to consume lots of sugar and fat that you're not intending to consume. Many muffins, for instance, are only about as healthy as a cupcake without frosting.

The recipes in this section, however, keep the sugar low and include protein. Just don't go crazy with the butter and syrup, and you'll keep these recipes nice and healthy.

Going gluten-free

If you have *celiac disease* (an allergy to gluten) or you're just sensitive to gluten, consider substituting the flour in these recipes for gluten-free flour.

You may have a gluten sensitivity if you have the following symptoms after eating gluten:

- Fatigue
- Bloating
- Gas
- Irritable bowel syndrome (IBS)
- Diarrhea
- Constipation
- Joint pain
- Migraines

- Mental fog
- Anxiety
- Depression
- Skin problems

And guess what else may be another symptom of gluten sensitivity? Acid reflux!

The average grocery store has several products for people who want to substitute gluten in their baked goods. Most combine several substitutes into one product, using ingredients such as potato starch, garbanzo flour, tapioca flour, sorghum flour, and fava flour. Several of those items include protein, which makes the baked good even healthier.

Fabulous French Toast

Prep time: 10 min • **Cook time:** 20 min • **Yield:** 4 servings

Ingredients	*Directions*
3 eggs	*1* In a large mixing bowl, add the eggs, milk, vanilla, cinnamon, and salt. Whisk until smooth.
1 cup lowfat milk	
1 teaspoon vanilla extract	*2* Heat a cast-iron skillet over medium heat.
½ teaspoon cinnamon	
Pinch of salt	*3* Soak the bread slices in the egg mixture until saturated, about 30 seconds each side.
8 slices 100 percent whole-grain bread, thickly sliced	*4* Cook in batches until the bread turns golden brown, about 4 minutes each side. Repeat until all the slices are cooked.
1 cup lowfat, plain yogurt	
1 banana, sliced	
1 tablespoon pure maple syrup	*5* Top the French toast with dollops of yogurt and bananas. Drizzle the maple syrup on top.

Per serving: Calories 322 (From Fat 66); Fat 7g (Saturated 3g); Cholesterol 146mg; Sodium 475mg; Carbohydrate 49g (Dietary Fiber 5g); Protein 17g.

Vary It! Not bananas for bananas? No problem! Any other type of fruit will taste good on this French toast. If you're not in the mood for fruit, try chopped nuts.

Pear Banana Nut Muffins

Prep time: 30 min • **Cook time:** 15–20 min • **Yield:** 12 servings

Ingredients	*Directions*
1 medium pear, peeled and diced	*1* Preheat the oven to 375 degrees. Line a 12-cup muffin pan with paper liners or grease the pan with olive oil; set aside.
2 tablespoons pear nectar	
1 cup whole-wheat flour	*2* In a 1-quart saucepan, combine the pear and pear nectar. Bring the mixture to a boil over medium heat. Reduce the heat to low and simmer for 3 minutes. Remove the pear mixture from the heat and mash it until it's smooth. Let the mixture cool for 15 minutes.
1 cup rolled oats	
1 tablespoon ground flaxseed	
3 tablespoons maple sugar flakes or Sucanat (optional)	*3* In a large bowl, combine the flour, oats, flaxseed, sugar flakes (if desired), baking powder, baking soda, cinnamon, cardamom, and sea salt. Mix well.
1 teaspoon baking powder	
½ teaspoon baking soda	
1 teaspoon cinnamon	*4* In a small bowl, combine the cooled pear mixture, eggs, almond milk, butter, vanilla, and banana; mix well.
¼ teaspoon cardamom	
¼ teaspoon sea salt	
2 eggs	*5* Add the pear mixture to the dry ingredients and stir just until combined. Stir in the walnuts. Spoon the batter into the prepared muffin pan.
⅓ cup vanilla almond milk	
2 tablespoons butter, melted	
2 teaspoons vanilla	*6* Bake for 15 to 20 minutes, or until the muffins are set and lightly browned. Remove the muffins from the pan and cool them on a wire rack.
1 medium banana, peeled and mashed	
1 cup chopped walnuts	

Per serving: Calories 180 (From Fat 92); Fat 10g (Saturated 2g); Cholesterol 41mg; Sodium 185mg; Carbohydrate 18g; Dietary Fiber 3g; Protein 5g.

Tip: To preserve the muffins' freshness, store them in an airtight container.

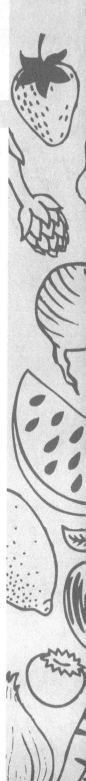

Banana Pecan Buckwheat Pancakes

Prep time: 30 min • **Cook time:** 20 min • **Yield:** 10–12 pancakes

Ingredients	Directions
³/₄ cup water	*1* In a medium bowl, mix the water, milk, salt, and 3 tablespoons of the oil.
1 cup soymilk or rice milk	
½ teaspoon sea salt	*2* In a large bowl, sift the flours and baking powder together.
4 tablespoons cold-pressed walnut or sesame oil, divided	
1³/₄ cups whole-wheat pastry flour	*3* Pour the wet ingredients into the dry ingredients and mix lightly with a whisk to a thick creamy consistency. Add a little more water if the batter is too thick.
¼ cup buckwheat flour	
1 tablespoon baking powder	*4* Chill the batter for 20 minutes, until it's cold.
½ cup chopped pecans	*5* In a skillet, dry-roast the pecans over medium heat for 5 to 7 minutes.
3 medium bananas, sliced	
Pure maple syrup, to taste	*6* Heat a heavy skillet over a high heat. Pour the remaining 1 tablespoon of oil into the skillet.
	7 Spoon ¼ cup of the batter into the skillet, add a few pieces of banana and some pecans, and cook until bubbles form on the top of the pancake.
	8 Flip the pancake and cook until it's lightly brown on both sides. Remove the pancake from the skillet, and repeat Steps 7 and 8 until you've used all the batter.
	9 Drizzle the pancakes with maple syrup before serving.

Per serving: Calories 163 (From Fat 59); Fat 7g (Saturated 1g); Cholesterol 0mg; Sodium 234mg; Carbohydrate 25g (Dietary Fiber 4g); Protein 4g.

Great Grains

One of the great things about grains is that they absorb the flavor of whatever you cook them with. They're begging for customization via fruit in your oatmeal, vanilla extract in your muesli, or cheese in your rice. There's no reason to eat bland granola or die-of-boredom grits. Flavor it up!

The recipes in this section do just that: They start with a healthy foundation of grain and then add other ingredients to liven it up. Grains are high in fiber and nutrients, including a host of B vitamins. We include several types of grains in these recipes, but there are many others including:

- ✔ Bulgur
- ✔ Rye
- ✔ Spelt
- ✔ Teff
- ✔ Titricale

Unless you have an allergy to a particular grain, every grain is a healthy food choice for the general population and for the acid-reflux sufferer. So, gain some grains with the following recipes.

The grains in this section are all wheat free! Although wheat is a perfectly healthy option for many people, it's one of the biggest offenders for people with gluten sensitivity.

Nut Butter Granola

Prep time: 15 min • **Cook time:** 35–45 min • **Yield:** 12 servings

Ingredients	Directions
4 cups rolled oats	**1** Preheat the oven to 300 degrees. Line a large baking sheet that has sides with parchment paper and set aside.
1 cup spelt flakes	
1 cup kamut flakes	
1 cup sliced raw almonds	**2** In a large bowl, combine the oats, spelt flakes, kamut flakes, almonds, wheat germ, flaxseeds (if desired), and sesame seeds; mix gently. Set aside.
⅓ cup wheat germ	
⅓ cup flaxseeds (optional)	
⅓ cup sesame seeds	**3** In a 1-quart saucepan, combine the nut butter, apple-sauce, butter, honey, cinnamon, and sea salt. Cook over low heat until the nut butter melts and the mixture combines. Remove the mixture from the heat and add the vanilla.
¾ cup almond or walnut butter	
½ cup unsweetened applesauce	
3 tablespoons butter, melted	**4** Pour the nut butter mixture over the mixed grains and nuts. Stir gently to coat; then spread evenly on the prepared baking sheet.
2 tablespoons raw honey	
2 teaspoons cinnamon	
½ teaspoon sea salt	**5** Bake the granola for 35 to 45 minutes, stirring every 10 minutes, until the granola is fragrant and lightly golden. Stir in the dried fruit and raisins.
2 teaspoons vanilla extract	
1 cup dried cranberries or cherries	
1 cup golden raisins	**6** Let the mixture cool for 1 hour, stirring every 15 minutes. Serve with yogurt, fresh fruit, or milk.

Per serving: Calories 321 (From Fat 102); Fat 11g (Saturated 3g); Cholesterol 8mg; Sodium 113mg; Carbohydrate 49g; Dietary Fiber 7g; Protein 9g.

Tip: To keep the granola fresh, store it in an airtight container.

Vary It! Any nut butter will work here. That includes, for instance, cashew butter, peanut butter, or hazelnut butter. Peanut butter will have the strongest flavor, which you may see as a good or bad thing.

Fast Morning Muesli

Prep time: 20 min • **Yield:** 4 servings

Ingredients	Directions
1 cup rolled oats	*1* In a large bowl, combine the oats and dates or raisins.
¼ cup dates or raisins	
3 cups soymilk or rice milk	*2* Cover the oats with milk. Stir in the vanilla extract, if desired.
1 teaspoon vanilla extract (optional)	
1 cup chopped almonds	*3* Leave the oats to soak for 15 to 20 minutes or overnight.
½ cup chopped walnuts	
½ cup sunflower seeds	*4* When ready to serve, stir in the almonds, walnuts, and sunflower seeds.

Per serving: Calories 417 (From Fat 238); Fat 27g (Saturated 3g); Cholesterol 0mg; Sodium 24mg; Carbohydrate 34g (Dietary Fiber 10g); Protein 17g.

Vary It! Soak the oats overnight in apple cider instead of milk.

Note: Muesli is common in Europe and a nice alternative to the mushiness of American-style oats.

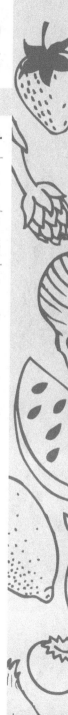

Winter Warming Oatmeal

Prep time: 5 min • **Cook time:** 20–25 min • **Yield:** 3–4 servings

Ingredients	Directions
4 cups water	**1** In a medium saucepan, add the water and sea salt. Cover and bring to a rolling boil.
⅛ to ¼ teaspoon sea salt	
1½ cups rolled oats	**2** Gently stir in the oats as you lower the heat to a simmer. Cover the pot about four-fifths to allow the steam to escape. Cook the oats for 10 to 15 minutes.
Handful of chopped roasted almonds	
2 tablespoons raisins	**3** Check occasionally to make sure the water hasn't evaporated. If the oats look dry, gently stir in ¼ to ½ cup of water. You may have to repeat this step if the heat is too high or if you want a creamier texture.
Pinch of cinnamon, or to taste	
	4 Add the almonds and raisins.
	5 Cook for another 10 minutes. Stir in the cinnamon and serve.

Per serving: Calories 481 (From Fat 247); Fat 27g (Saturated 2g); Cholesterol 0mg; Sodium 113mg; Carbohydrate 47g (Dietary Fiber 10g); Protein 18g.

Tip: To get a creamy consistency, cook the oats longer while continuously adding small amounts of water until you reach the desired consistency.

Tip: Almonds are usually available already toasted at natural food stores. For a nuttier flavor, you can chop and dry-roast the nuts in a skillet over medium-low heat for approximately 15 minutes, or until they turn slightly brown, and then add them to the oatmeal.

Vary It! Mixing in ingredients like roasted seeds or nuts, a pinch of salt, or whatever else suits your fancy adds variety to this standard breakfast.

Southern-Style Corn Grits

Prep time: 8 min • **Cook time:** 9 min • **Yield:** 4 servings

Ingredients	Directions
1 cup corn grits	**1** In a small bowl, whisk together the corn grits with 1½ cups of the water; let it stand for 3 minutes.
3 cups water	
¼ teaspoon sea salt	**2** In a medium saucepan, bring the remaining 1½ cups of water to a boil.
1 cup chopped walnuts	
Pure maple syrup, to taste	**3** Pour the grits into the boiling water. Add the salt.
	4 Reduce the heat to low, and stir the grits vigorously until they become thick and creamy.
	5 In a skillet, dry-roast the walnuts over medium-low heat for 3 to 4 minutes.
	6 Stir the walnuts into the grits. Divide into 4 bowls and drizzle with maple syrup before serving.

Per serving: Calories 367 (From Fat 181); Fat 20g (Saturated 2g); Cholesterol 0mg; Sodium 147mg; Carbohydrate 42g (Dietary Fiber 3g); Protein 8g.

Note: What the heck are grits, anyway? People seem to either love grits, or fear them. *Grits* isn't the most fortunate moniker, after all. This Southern staple is a warm dish of ground corn, a little like a soft polenta. Grits are porridge-like and accept flavor well, such as from salt, pepper, herbs, and cheese.

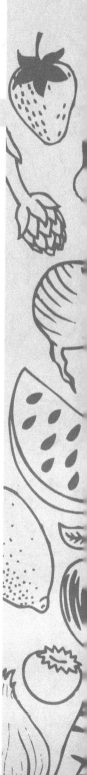

Rice and Shine

Prep time: 10 min • **Cook time:** 10 min • **Yield:** 4 servings

Ingredient	Directions
3 cups cooked brown rice	**1** In a saucepan, combine all the ingredients.
¾ cup lowfat milk	
½ cup raisins	**2** Cook on medium heat until the ingredients are mixed well and warm throughout.
½ cup applesauce	
¼ cup walnut pieces	
2 tablespoons honey	
1 teaspoon cinnamon	
Pinch of salt	

Per serving: Calories 341 (From Fat 53); Fat 6g (Saturated 1g); Cholesterol 2mg; Sodium 68mg; Carbohydrate 66g (Dietary Fiber 5g); Protein 7g.

Morning Millet

Prep time: 10 min • **Cook time:** 4–8 hr • **Yield:** 4 servings

Ingredients	Directions
½ cup millet	**1** In a 3½-quart slow cooker, add the millet, almond milk, fruit, and salt.
2 cups vanilla almond milk	
3 peaches or nectarines, cored, pitted, and chopped	**2** Cook for 4 hours on high or 8 hours on low.
⅛ teaspoon salt	**3** Mix well and serve warm in a bowl.
2 tablespoons pumpkin seeds, for garnish	**4** Garnish with pumpkin seeds.

Per serving: Calories 197 (From Fat 42); Fat 5g (Saturated 1g); Cholesterol 0mg; Sodium 145mg; Carbohydrate 35g (Dietary Fiber 4g); Protein 14g.

Vary It! Frozen peaches or nectarines will also work if you don't have fresh. If you use frozen, use 2 cups.

How to prepare pumpkin seeds

You can buy precooked, salted pumpkin seeds. Or you can buy raw pumpkin seeds and leave them just the way they are.

If you want more flavor, though, you can take those raw pumpkin seeds, spread them onto a baking sheet, spritz them with water from a spray bottle, and then sprinkle with salt. Bake on low heat (325 degrees or lower) until golden brown. Stir the seeds halfway through the cook time.

To start from scratch, buy a pumpkin. Cut the top off, and scoop the mush out of the pumpkin. Separate the seeds from the goo. Put the seeds in a strainer and wash thoroughly. Spread onto a baking sheet, sprinkle with salt, and follow the directions above.

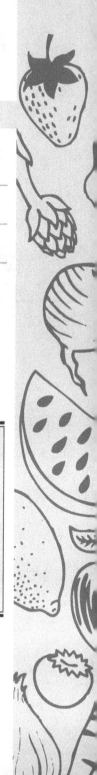

Fruits and Veggies

There's a really easy way to get fruits and veggies in your diet: Eat an apple, or make a serving of sautéed broccoli, or eat a banana, or cook up some zucchini, or munch on some carrot sticks. All right, you get the drift. Eating fruits and veggies in their whole state is a wonderful way to get the nutrients in a balanced way.

If you juice a pear, that juice is still healthy, but it lacks the balance of fiber that it had when you separated the juice from the fruit itself. Without the fiber, the body digests the sugar more quickly, and that means the juice is more likely to spike your blood sugar than if you'd absorbed the fruit in its whole state.

"Messing" with fruits and veggies by juicing them, cooking them, or combining them with other ingredients can still be a great and healthy choice, but always remember that a plain-old whole apple, or a handful of grapes, or some celery sticks, is the best for you, is good for your reflux, and is easier than any recipe.

That said, the recipes in this section are about as easy as they get. Quick and healthy. Each of these recipes can be made the night before, but keep in mind that there will be more nutrients if you consume the food soon after making it instead of after it's been in the refrigerator for ten hours.

Great Green Smoothies

Prep time: 8 min • **Yield:** 2 servings

Ingredients	Directions
1 cucumber	**1** Trim the ends of the cucumber, and cut the remaining section into 6 pieces.
½ cup parsley	
1 apple, cored and sliced	**2** Add all the ingredients to a blender, and blend until smooth.
1 avocado, cored and peeled	
4 cups raw baby spinach	
One 1-inch cube fresh ginger, peeled	
3 cups coconut water	
10 ice cubes	

Per serving: Calories 279 (From Fat 104); Fat 12g (Saturated 1g); Cholesterol 0mg; Sodium 108mg; Carbohydrate 44g (Dietary Fiber 9g); Protein 6g.

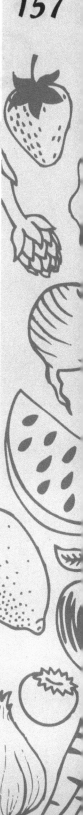

How to cut an avocado

Choose avocados that are *not* rock hard. They should have a little give when you buy them, or be soft (but not mushy). If you can only find avocados that are hard, put them in the sun or in a paper bag on the counter. Don't refrigerate unless the avocado is already ripe.

When it's ripe, you're ready to go. Cut the avocado lengthwise. Scoop the seed out with a spoon or stick a knife into it and pull it out that way. Score the meat with a knife one way, then the other, so the "meat" is diced. Use a tablespoon to scoop the meat out from each half of the peel. Scrape the peel to get as much of the green stuff as possible. (See the figure for an illustration of this process.)

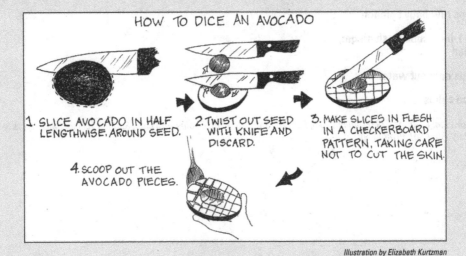

HOW TO DICE AN AVOCADO

1. SLICE AVOCADO IN HALF LENGTHWISE, AROUND SEED.

2. TWIST OUT SEED WITH KNIFE AND DISCARD.

3. MAKE SLICES IN FLESH IN A CHECKERBOARD PATTERN, TAKING CARE NOT TO CUT THE SKIN.

4. SCOOP OUT THE AVOCADO PIECES.

Illustration by Elizabeth Kurtzman

Cantaloupe Banana Smoothies

Prep time: 5 min • **Yield:** 4 servings

Ingredients	Directions
2 cups peeled, cubed cantaloupe	**1** In a blender or food processor, combine the cantaloupe, banana, orange juice, and lemon juice. Cover and blend on high until the fruits are well mixed.
1 banana, peeled, cut into chunks, and frozen	
½ cup orange juice	**2** Add the yogurt, flaxseeds, and vanilla. Cover and blend on high until the mixture is smooth. Divide the smoothie evenly into 4 glasses and serve immediately.
1 tablespoon lemon juice	
1 cup organic yogurt	
1 tablespoon flaxseeds	
1 teaspoon vanilla	

Per serving: Calories 121 (From Fat 28); Fat 3g (Saturated 1g); Cholesterol 8mg; Sodium 36mg; Carbohydrate 21g; Dietary Fiber 2g; Protein 4g.

Vary It! You can switch up this simple recipe in many ways. For example, use honeydew melon in place of the cantaloupe or add a peeled, sliced peach or pear to the mix.

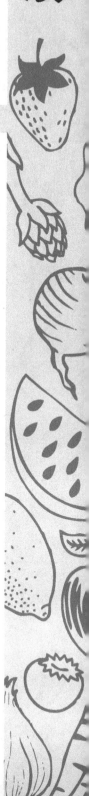

Fruit Salad with Yogurt

Prep time: 15 min • **Yield:** 2 servings

Ingredients	*Directions*
1 tablespoon chia seeds (optional)	*1* In a large bowl, stir the chia seeds into the yogurt until mixed well.
1 cup lowfat plain yogurt	
½ cantaloupe, cut into bite-size pieces	*2* Add the remaining ingredients to the bowl and mix until the fruit is coated with yogurt.
10 grapes, cut in half	
½ banana, cut into 1/8-inch slices	*3* Drizzle with maple syrup. Eat immediately before it thickens.
3 strawberries, cut into halves	
¼ cup fresh or frozen blueberries	
2 tablespoons pure maple syrup	

Per serving: Calories 238 (From Fat 21); Fat 2g (Saturated 1g); Cholesterol 7mg; Sodium 111mg; Carbohydrate 49g (Dietary Fiber 3g); Protein 8g.

Greek yogurt: The king of yogurts

Although you can find many yogurts lining the shelves of your local grocery store, lowfat plain Greek yogurt reigns over the rest. One reason: All the liquid whey is drained out, leaving a thicker, creamier texture. Face it: Creamier is just better!

Along with the normal health benefits of yogurt (such as calcium, potassium, and vitamins B6 and B12), Greek yogurt contains twice the protein of regular yogurt, keeping you feeling fuller longer. Greek yogurt is also lower in sugar and higher in the probiotic cultures that are helpful for healthy digestion. Choose lowfat plain Greek yogurt to save on fat grams and calories. If you aren't used to the taste of plain yogurt, mix in some all-fruit spread or fresh berries to add a little sweetness.

Chapter 10

Fulfilling Lunches

*I*f you eat the wrong type of lunch (for instance, a monstrous burrito full of red meat, onions, chili peppers, and hot sauce), you may feel so bad that you throw in the towel and eat a dinner that just prolongs the misery. The recipes in this chapter will keep you on the right path. They're healthy and easy, and they should give you a break from reflux while you take a break from school or work to have that important midday meal.

Succulent Salads

There's a big disparity in salad quality out there. In the past, many people thought of a "salad" as a handful of iceberg lettuce, a tomato wedge, and dressing. As the foodie movement continues, people are starting to expect more from their salads. More impressive salads have bases of spinach, arugula, spring mix, or other greens, and incorporate fruits, toasted nuts, raw nuts, creative dressings, choice meats, and every cheese you can name. These gourmet salads aren't new — they're just more prevalent than before.

Beware the salad that looks healthy but is loaded with calories. Clues that your salad may not be a great choice: lots of bacon, croutons, thick fatty dressing, and fists full of cheese.

The salads in this section are very different from each other, so you'll have one for every type of meal, whether you want something hearty or light.

Salmon and New Potato Salad

Prep time: 15 min • **Cook time:** 20 min • **Yield:** 4 servings

Ingredients	Directions
1 pound red new potatoes, scrubbed	*1* Preheat the oven to 400 degrees.
1 pound wild salmon filet	*2* In a large saucepan, place the potatoes and add water to cover. Bring to a boil over high heat, reduce the heat to medium-low, cover, and simmer until the potatoes are tender when pierced with a fork, about 15 minutes. Drain the water from the potatoes and cut into quarters.
Salt and pepper, to taste	
4 tablespoons olive oil	
3 tablespoons balsamic vinegar	
8 cups packed baby salad greens	*3* Meanwhile, in a large baking pan, place the salmon filet and season with salt and pepper. Roast for 10 to 12 minutes, until the fish is flaky. Transfer the salmon to a plate and cut into 1-inch chunks. Remove the skin.
1 tablespoon fresh basil, chopped	
	4 In a small jar, combine the oil and vinegar. Shake until well blended.
	5 In a large bowl, gently toss the salad greens and basil with the dressing. Add the salmon and potatoes, and toss enough to coat with dressing. Enjoy immediately.

Per serving: Calories 440 (From Fat 195); Fat 22g (Saturated 3g); Cholesterol 72mg; Sodium 286mg; Carbohydrate 28g (Dietary Fiber 4g); Protein 30g.

Vary It! Not crazy about new potatoes? No worries! Use a different type of potato. Any type will do. You can also use more than one kind of potato. Using colored potatoes (purple, red, Yukon gold) can make your salad look especially appetizing.

Pasta Salad

Prep time: 15 min • **Cook time:** 10 min • **Yield:** 4 servings

Ingredients	Directions
One 12-ounce package cheese-filled tortellini	*1* In a large saucepan, cook the pasta according to the package instructions. Add the broccoli and carrot to the saucepan in the last 4 minutes. Drain the pasta and vegetables.
3 cups broccoli florets, chopped	
1 large carrot, thinly sliced	*2* Meanwhile, in a small bowl, whisk together the vinegar, olive oil, basil, mustard, oregano, and salt and pepper.
½ cup white wine vinegar	
2 tablespoons olive oil	
2 tablespoons fresh basil, chopped	*3* In a large salad bowl, combine the pasta mixture with the beans, bell pepper, and olives.
2 tablespoons Dijon mustard	
1 teaspoon oregano, dried	*4* Pour the vinegar mixture over the pasta and mix until the pasta is evenly coated.
Salt and pepper, to taste	
4 ounces canned kidney beans, drained	
1 large red bell pepper, chopped	
¼ cup black olives, sliced	

Per serving: Calories 409 (From Fat 129); Fat 14g (Saturated 4g); Cholesterol 36mg; Sodium 820mg; Carbohydrate 55g (Dietary Fiber 7g); Protein 16g.

Vary It! Almost any ingredient can go in this recipe. Extra vegetables, more beans, some meat, cheese . . . throw it in! Just keep your reflux in mind. So, no red meat, not too much cheese (because excess fat makes reflux worse), and no onions, peppers, tomatoes, or citrus.

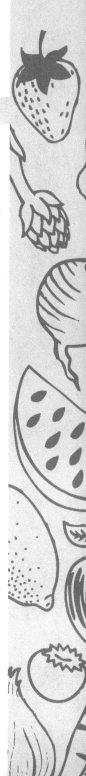

Fruity Chicken Pasta Salad

Prep time: 15 min, plus refrigerating time • **Cook time:** 10 min • **Yield:** 6 servings

Ingredients	*Directions*
½ cup lowfat Greek or regular yogurt	**1** In a large bowl, combine the yogurt, sour cream, buttermilk or almond milk, vinegar, mustard, honey, thyme, sea salt, and white pepper; mix well to blend.
¼ cup lowfat sour cream	
3 tablespoons buttermilk or almond milk	**2** In a large saucepan, cook the pasta according to the package directions, until the pasta is just tender. Drain well and add the pasta to the bowl with the dressing from Step 1.
2 tablespoons apple cider vinegar	
2 tablespoons mustard	
2 tablespoons raw honey	**3** Stir in the chicken and celery until they're well coated. Gently add the grapes, blueberries, cantaloupe, and walnuts. Stir gently. Cover and refrigerate for 2 to 3 hours before serving.
1 teaspoon dried thyme	
½ teaspoon sea salt	
⅛ teaspoon white pepper	
4 cups whole-wheat penne or farfalle pasta	
3 cups cooked chicken, cut into 1-inch pieces	
3 stalks celery, sliced	
2 cups red grapes	
1 cup blueberries	
2 cups cubed cantaloupe	
½ cup walnut pieces	

Per serving: Calories 492 (From Fat 129); Fat 14g (Saturated 3g); Cholesterol 68mg; Sodium 439mg; Carbohydrate 67g (Dietary Fiber 8g); Protein 31g.

Crunchy Boiled Salad with Pumpkin Seed Dressing

Prep time: 10 min • **Cook time:** 10 min • **Yield:** 4 servings

Ingredients	Directions
¼ cup carrots, cut into diagonals	**1** In a medium saucepan, bring 1½ to 2 inches of water to a boil.
1 cup snow peas	**2** Place the carrots in a steamer basket and steam over the boiling water for 2 to 3 minutes. Remove and place in a mixing bowl.
¼ cup red radishes, cut into quarters	
1 cup broccoli florets	**3** Repeat Step 2 with the snow peas, adding them to the mixing bowl with the carrots after they're steamed. Repeat with the radishes and the broccoli.
1 tablespoon fresh parsley	
Pumpkin Seed Dressing (see the following recipe)	**4** Add the parsley to the mixing bowl with the vegetables.
	5 Drizzle the Pumpkin Seed Dressing over the vegetables, toss lightly, and serve.

Pumpkin Seed Dressing

1 tablespoon pumpkin seeds	**1** Toast the pumpkin seeds in a small skillet over medium heat until brown.
1 tablespoon shoyu (or tamari)	
1 tablespoon water	**2** In a small saucepan, combine the shoyu and water and simmer over low heat for 3 minutes.
1 tablespoon grated fresh ginger	
1 tablespoon honey	**3** Remove the pan from the heat. Add the ginger, honey, and pumpkin seeds, and stir well.

Per serving: Calories 50 (From Fat 10); Fat 1g (Saturated 0g); Cholesterol 0mg; Sodium 255mg; Carbohydrate 9g (Dietary Fiber 2g); Protein 2g.

Vary It! Boiled salad is a super-delicious alternative to a lettuce-based salad. You can use whatever is in your fridge and as little or as many vegetables as you like. The idea is to lightly cook the vegetables in the same water, starting with blander vegetables and working up to the stronger flavors.

Cobb Salad with Vinaigrette

Prep time: 10 min • **Yield:** 6 servings

Ingredients

10 ounces spinach leaves, chopped

3 eggs, hardboiled, peeled, and chopped into small pieces

1 medium tomato, chopped

1 to 2 avocados, stones removed, flesh scooped out of shell, and sliced

10 ripe black olives, pitted and finely chopped

¼ to ½ cup grated cheddar cheese

¼ cup bacon bits

Vinaigrette (see the following recipe)

Directions

1 In a salad bowl, toss together the spinach, eggs, tomato, and avocado.

2 Sprinkle the top of the salad with the olives, cheese, and bacon bits. Toss with the Vinaigrette.

Vinaigrette

8 teaspoons olive oil

2 to 3 tablespoons mock (young) balsamic vinegar

1½ teaspoons red wine vinegar

1½ teaspoons ground mustard

1½ teaspoons honey

⅛ teaspoon salt, or to taste

⅛ teaspoon pepper, or to taste

In a small bowl, combine all the ingredients thoroughly until they dissolve into each other.

Per serving: Calories 214 (From Fat 141); Fat 16g (Saturated 4g); Cholesterol 101mg; Sodium 391mg; Carbohydrate 12g (Dietary Fiber 4g); Protein 9g.

Sandwiches and Wraps

Where would we be without the sandwich? This mainstay of Western culinary culture appears in other cuisines as well, just not as prevalently. Any time ingredients are rolled or stuffed into a breadlike food, a sandwich is born. So, the sandwich is as old as bread.

Bread itself adds a lot to the taste and overall enjoyment of a sandwich, but bread is also a matter of convenience because it makes the contents so much easier to eat, and makes it all travel better. What's peanut butter and jelly without bread? Er, peanut butter and jelly. Bread please!

There are accounts of ancient Jews wrapping lamb meat and herbs between soft *matzo* (unleavened bread) during Passover. Sounds like a sandwich. And in many other cultures, including Indian, Middle Eastern, and African, people use small pieces of bread to scoop food, such as thick porridges of vegetable or meat. That's like a tiny sandwich in every bite. The aforementioned cultures still use bread in this way, from pita to *injera* (an Ethiopian bread similar to a crêpe). The tortilla has also been used in a similar way for many generations.

The sandwich has existed for thousands of years, but according to legend, it wasn't called a "sandwich" until John Montagu, the Fourth Earl of Sandwich, dubbed it such. Who says the British haven't contributed anything worthwhile to gastronomy?

If you're not big on bread or you want to switch up a sandwich you're getting tired of, try a wrap. Wraps aren't new, but they are becoming more popular. In the 1990s, when carbs were considered as desirable as taxes, people wanted to minimize bread as much as possible. Because wraps almost always use tortillas or very thin bread, wraps were a good solution to cutting down on bread.

If you have a gluten sensitivity or you're flat-out allergic to gluten, you've probably already discovered stores near you where you can buy gluten-free bread. If you haven't, give it a shot. These products are becoming widespread. Rice bread, for instance, can be used in place of any white or wheat sandwich bread. Gluten-free bread is usually harder than other sliced sandwich bread and can be a little bland, but it's still effective for the acid reflux–friendly recipes in this section.

Terrific Turkey Wraps

Prep time: 15 min • **Yield:** 4 servings

Ingredients	Directions
One 8-ounce package cream cheese	**1** In a medium bowl, mix the cream cheese, walnuts, celery, honey, and salt and pepper.
¼ cup walnuts, chopped	
¼ cup celery, finely chopped	**2** Divide the cream cheese mixture among the tortillas and spread it evenly.
2 tablespoons honey	
Salt and pepper, to taste	**3** Divide the cranberry sauce among the tortillas and spread it on top of the cream cheese.
Four 12-inch whole-wheat tortillas	
½ cup cranberry sauce, jellied	**4** Divide the turkey among the tortillas and place it on top of the cranberry sauce.
10 ounces roasted turkey, thinly sliced	
4 pieces green-leaf lettuce	**5** Add lettuce to each tortilla.
	6 Fold up the bottom of each tortilla and roll it like a burrito.

Per serving: Calories 569 (From Fat 539); Fat 30g (Saturated 12g); Cholesterol 121mg; Sodium 722mg; Carbohydrate 50g (Dietary Fiber 3g); Protein 31g.

Vary It! Roasted turkey isn't the only choice here. However, the cranberry sauce does preclude you from certain choices. For instance, cranberry sauce and crabmeat? No, thanks! Chicken or duck will work perfectly well, as long as you don't mind deviating from the Thanksgiving theme.

Veggie Pitas

Prep time: 20 min • **Yield:** 4 servings

Ingredients	Directions
1 cup plain yogurt	**1** In a small bowl, mix the yogurt, chopped cucumber, and dill.
1 small cucumber, half chopped, half sliced	
1 teaspoon dried dill	**2** In a food processor, add the beans, olives, olive oil, and salt and pepper. Mix until well blended and smooth.
1 cup garbanzo beans, drained	
5 Kalamata olives	
2 tablespoons extra-virgin olive oil	**3** Cut the pitas in half. Line one side of the inner part of each pita with the yogurt mixture and the other side with the bean mixture.
Salt and pepper, to taste	
2 whole-wheat pitas	**4** Fill the center of each pita with the sliced cucumber, bell pepper, and spinach.
½ small red bell pepper, sliced	
1 cup baby spinach	

Per serving: Calories 259 (From Fat 92); Fat 10g (Saturated 2g); Cholesterol 4mg; Sodium 563mg; Carbohydrate 34g (Dietary Fiber 5g); Protein 10g.

Tip: There's a Mediterranean theme to this recipe, and that's for good reason: Most Mediterranean food is healthy, and this cuisine can be a good choice for people trying to reduce reflux. Just avoid the onions, garlic, and tomatoes that can be prevalent in Mediterranean fare, and you'll be fine.

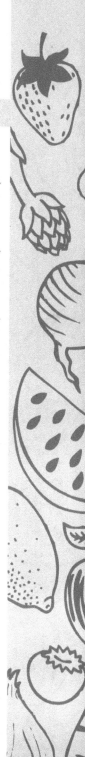

Tofu Sandwiches

Prep time: 15 min • **Cook time:** 20 min • **Yield:** 4 servings

Ingredients	Directions
1 to 2 tablespoons Dijon mustard	**1** Preheat the oven to 475 degrees.
1 tablespoon reduced-sodium soy sauce	**2** In a small bowl, combine the mustard and soy sauce.
12 ounces extra-firm tofu, drained and rinsed	**3** Slice the tofu crosswise into eight ½-inch-thick pieces. Pat dry with a paper towel and place on a greased baking sheet.
1 avocado, peeled, pitted, and sliced	**4** Using a spoon, cover both sides of the tofu with the mustard mixture.
4 pieces green-leaf lettuce	
8 slices whole-wheat bread, toasted	**5** Bake the tofu for 30 minutes.
	6 Divide the avocado, lettuce, and tofu among 4 slices of the toast and top with the remaining toast to make 4 sandwiches.
	7 Cut the sandwiches in half.

Per serving: Calories 304 (From Fat 109); Fat 12g (Saturated 2g); Cholesterol 0mg; Sodium 526mg; Carbohydrate 34g (Dietary Fiber 5g); Protein 17g.

Note: Tofu scares some people, but it shouldn't. It doesn't look great unprepared, but neither does chicken when you think about it. Tofu is white and usually in a brick shape about 2 inches tall, 3 inches wide, and 5 inches deep. It's typically packed in water inside a plastic carton. You can find tofu in the refrigerated section of most grocery stores. On its own, tofu has almost no flavor, which means it can pick up almost any flavor you pair it with. So, cover it with sauce, marinate it, or sauté it with flavors you like.

Savory Soups

It's a cold winter day. It's dark and gloomy. Your heater is on full blast and you're under an electric blanket, but the chill is still in your bones. And you're hungry! What do you want to eat: A salad or a hot bowl of soup? Soup!

Soup is great fresh, but it also tastes good the next day, and the day after that. Many soups taste even better after they've sat — a day or two in the fridge can really bring out the flavor. Soup freezes well, too. Certain soups can be labor and/or time intensive, but that initial investment can be well worth it if you make a big enough pot of it. And then there are soups that are "souper" easy (pardon the pun).

Soups can be tricky for people with acid reflux, because most soups rely on a base that's heavy on onions. This base, a *mirepoix,* is a rough chop of onions, celery, and carrots, and sometimes includes garlic. *Mirepoix* is a French creation, and it's hard to avoid when you eat out, because it isn't in the ingredient list on menus. However, a cup or even a bowl of soup with a *mirepoix* base probably won't bother your reflux if the other ingredients are reflux friendly enough.

Obvious soups to avoid are tomato soup (if tomatoes are one of your triggers), and French onion soup. Mexican soups can have triggers, too, so ask the cook what's in the soup and take small portions — if you do well, have a bigger portion next time you visit that restaurant.

Soup consistency is very particular, so if any of the soups in this book are too thick for your taste, thin them out a little with water, chicken stock, or vegetable stock. Soups get thicker as they sit, so if you make enough for leftovers, you'll probably have to thin it out when you reheat it anyway. Either way, thick or thin, the soup recipes in this chapter should help keep your reflux away.

Borscht (Beet Soup)

Prep time: 10 min • **Cook time:** 45 min • **Yield:** 8 servings

Ingredients	*Directions*
Two 32-ounce containers chicken broth	1 In a large pot, bring the chicken broth to a boil and then add the potatoes. Boil for 3 minutes if the potatoes are grated and 5 minutes if the potatoes are in chunks. Add the cabbage to the pot and boil for another 5 minutes.
2 medium potatoes, chopped into small squares or grated	
1/3 cup red or green cabbage, grated or chopped	
1 tablespoon olive oil	2 Put the olive oil in a medium pot, add the carrots, and stir occasionally for 2 to 3 minutes.
2 carrots, grated	
5 medium beets, grated	3 Put the beets into the pot with the carrots and cook for 1 minute. Then add the tomato and stir-fry for another 1 minute. Add the parsley, dill, and bay leaf and stir for another minute.
1 tomato, blanched and chopped coarsely	
1 tablespoon fresh parsley or 1 tablespoon dried parsley	4 Throw everything into the pot with the chicken broth, and simmer for about 30 minutes.
1 tablespoon fresh dill or 1 teaspoon dried dill	
1 bay leaf	5 Serve when the vegetables are tender (making sure to remove the bay leaf).

Per serving: Calories 98 (From Fat 27); Fat 3g (Saturated 0g); Cholesterol 0mg; Sodium 1,072mg; Carbohydrate 15g (Dietary Fiber 2g); Protein 3g.

Tip: Do you like your soup chunky? Leave it as is. If you want your soup smooth, puree it right in the pot with a hand blender. Craving a creamy soup? In a bowl, mix a 12-ounce package of soft tofu with a cup of the broth, puree it with a hand blender, and add it to the broth after it has simmered for 20 minutes.

Tip: If you're going to grate the veggies in this recipe, using a decent food processor will save you grated knuckles and loads of time. Grate the beets first and empty them into a bowl. Repeat the process with the carrots, the potatoes, and then the cabbage. Don't bother cleaning the grater in between. If you have a little beet mixed in with the cabbage, it'll boil longer, which is great; you just don't want the cabbage to get mixed in and boil less.

Carrot Ginger Soup

Prep time: 20 min • **Yield:** 4 servings

Ingredients	Directions
3 cups carrot juice	**1** In a blender, place the carrot juice, avocados, salt, and ginger and blend on high until smooth.
2 ripe avocados, peeled and pitted	
1½ teaspoons salt	**2** Taste and add more ginger or salt if desired.
1 teaspoon peeled and grated ginger	**3** Pour into bowls, top with diced avocado or crème fraîche, and serve.
Diced avocado or crème fraîche, for serving	

Per serving: Calories 178 (From Fat 101); Fat 11g (Saturated 1g); Cholesterol 0mg; Sodium 992mg; Carbohydrate 19g (Dietary Fiber 3g); Protein 4g.

Note: This soup will keep in the refrigerator for 5 days; avoid freezing it.

Vary It! For a sweeter taste to your soup, add 1 tablespoon agave nectar.

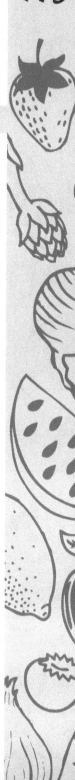

Lentil Soup

Prep time: 15 min • **Cook time:** 1 hr 15 min • **Yield:** 6 servings

Ingredients	*Directions*
¼ cup olive oil	*1* In a large pot, heat the oil over medium heat. Add the carrots, celery, and zucchini to the pot and cook until the vegetables are tender.
2 carrots	
2 stalks celery, chopped	
1 medium zucchini, chopped	*2* Add the oregano, basil, and bay leaf to the pot and cook for another 3 minutes.
1 teaspoon dried oregano	
1 teaspoon dried basil	*3* Add the lentils and vegetable broth to the pot and bring to a boil. Reduce the heat and simmer for 1 hour.
1 bay leaf	
2 cups dry lentils	
8 cups low-sodium vegetable broth	*4* Prior to serving, add the spinach, parsley, and vinegar to the lentils and cook until wilted.
½ cup spinach, rinsed and loosely chopped	*5* Add the salt and pepper.
½ cup Italian parsley, rinsed and loosely chopped	
1 tablespoon balsamic vinegar	
Salt and pepper, to taste	

Per serving: Calories 345 (From Fat 87); Fat 10g (Saturated 1g); Cholesterol 0mg; Sodium 337mg; Carbohydrate 47g (Dietary Fiber 17g); Protein 18g.

Note: Lentils are an extremely popular food around the world, which is great, because they're very healthy! Humans have been eating lentils for 9,000 to 13,000 years! In the United States, brown lentils are the most common form, but they also come in yellow, orange, green, and black varieties.

Culture Cuisine

Culture cuisine, like *ethnic cuisine,* is a tough term to pin down. Every food comes from some culture or some ethnicity. Many white Americans tend to use the term *ethnic food* for anything that isn't roast beef, mashed potatoes, and gravy. It's certainly faster to say, "Do you want to get ethnic food tonight?" than it is to say, "Do you want to get some kind of food that's different from what we usually eat? Some kind of food from another country, or from a culture in our country that we're not a member of?"

Food from some cultures is friendlier for sufferers of acid reflux than food from other cultures, but every culture has reflux-friendly options. Just be on the lookout for trigger foods (see Chapter 4) and avoid dishes that include them.

To find out more about which cultural cuisines are easiest for people with acid reflux and which ones are toughest, see Chapter 15. The most difficult trigger food to avoid in all cultural cuisine? Onions.

You'll be safe with the options in this section. Just be careful with the salsa you may want to put on the tacos — try making your own and going very light on the onions and garlic. You may want to forgo adding salsa all together. Some slices of avocado with a little salt may give the tacos that extra something you're looking for, even though avocado tastes very different from salsa.

Black Bean Tacos

Prep time: 10 min • **Cook time:** 8 min • **Yield:** 4 servings

Ingredients	Directions
One 15-ounce can black beans, drained	**1** In a medium saucepan, heat the beans, chilies, zucchini, cilantro, cumin, and salt and pepper on medium heat until warm throughout.
One 4-ounce can mild green chilies	
½ small zucchini, chopped	**2** Warm the tortillas in the microwave for 10 to 30 seconds, until soft and pliable.
2 tablespoons chopped fresh cilantro	
½ teaspoon cumin	**3** Spoon the bean mixture onto the tortillas.
Salt and pepper, to taste	**4** Top the bean mixture with the cheese and cabbage.
Eight 6-inch corn tortillas	
½ cup cheddar cheese, shredded	**5** Softly fold the tortillas in half.
1 cup green cabbage, shredded and seasoned with a pinch of salt and pepper	

Per serving: Calories 246 (From Fat 59); Fat 7g (Saturated 3g); Cholesterol 0mg; Sodium 663mg; Carbohydrate 37g (Dietary Fiber 8g); Protein 11g.

Vary It! Pinto beans will work just as well as black beans in this recipe, so give those a shot instead if they're your preference.

Steak Peanut Saté

Prep time: 5 min • **Cook time:** 10 min • **Yield:** 4 servings

Ingredients	Directions
8 ounces top sirloin steak	**1** Cut the steak into ¼-inch slices.
1 teaspoon toasted sesame oil	
2 teaspoons tamari	**2** Add the oil to a large skillet. Sauté the steak slices in the oil over medium heat for about 4 minutes.
1 tablespoon natural peanut butter	
1 teaspoon Dijon mustard	**3** Dissolve the tamari, peanut butter, and mustard in the water and pour the mixture over the steak.
½ cup water	
2 cups mustard greens or bok choy	**4** Add the greens and peanuts, cover, and simmer over medium heat for 5 minutes.
3 tablespoon roasted peanuts	**5** Turn off the heat and mix in the sprouts, if desired. The heat from the other ingredients will cook the sprouts.
1 cup bean sprouts (optional)	
	6 Serve with noodles or in a pita.

Per serving: Calories 177 (From Fat 101); Fat 11g (Saturated 3g); Cholesterol 37mg; Sodium 268mg; Carbohydrate 4g (Dietary Fiber 2g); Protein 16g.

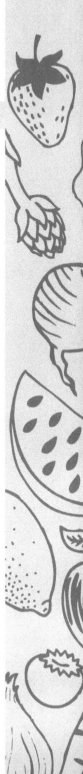

Chapter 11

Delectable Dinners

In This Chapter

▶ Ending your day the reflux-friendly way

▶ Finding a variety of dinners to please any palate

Dinner is a tough meal for people with acid reflux who like to consume a bulk of their calories at night. Eating too much food puts pressure on the lower esophageal sphincter (LES), and that pressure can activate reflux. Keep your dinner portions moderate, and you're less likely to get reflux.

Great Grains

Grains are an integral part of every culture's cuisine. They're full of fiber (as long as they're not overly processed) and nutrients and grains are extremely economical.

The most common way to cook grains is to boil or simmer them. To reduce cook time, soak the grains overnight.

Grains pick up flavor very well, so consider cooking them in stock or otherwise flavored water if you want them to have extra flavor. A rice cooker is helpful for — you guessed it — rice, but a good old-fashioned pot will do the trick just as well.

Dry grains store well for years, but be sure to store them in jars with the lid on tight or in Tupperware containers. These storage methods will keep grains safer from critters than a bag or box.

Chicken and Brown Rice Risotto

Prep time: 20 min • **Cook time:** 1 hr 10 • **Yield:** 6 servings

Ingredients	*Directions*
6 cups chicken stock	*1* In a medium saucepan, heat the chicken stock over low heat.
2 tablespoons olive oil	
2 tablespoons butter	*2* In a 3-quart saucepan, combine the olive oil with 1 tablespoon of the butter over medium heat. Add the chicken thighs and mushrooms; sprinkle with the sea salt. Cook and stir until the mushrooms are tender, about 5 to 6 minutes.
4 boneless, skinless chicken thighs, cubed	
1 cup chopped cremini mushrooms	
½ teaspoon sea salt	*3* Add the rice; cook and stir for 4 minutes.
1½ cups short- or medium-grain brown rice	*4* Add ½ cup of the chicken stock; cook, stirring frequently, until the stock is absorbed, about 4 minutes. Reduce the heat to low.
1 cup frozen peas, thawed	
½ cup grated Parmesan cheese	*5* Continue adding stock in ½-cup portions, stirring frequently. Add more stock as it's absorbed until the rice is tender, about 50 to 55 minutes.
¼ cup chopped flat-leaf parsley	
2 tablespoons chopped fresh basil	*6* Stir in the peas; cook for 2 minutes.
	7 Add the Parmesan cheese and the remaining 1 tablespoon of butter; cook for 2 to 3 minutes until the cheese and butter are melted.
	8 Add the parsley and basil and stir. Serve immediately.

Per serving: Calories 448 (From Fat 167); Fat 19g (Saturated 6g); Cholesterol 120mg; Sodium 1,306mg; Carbohydrate 41g (Dietary Fiber 3g); Protein 27g.

Tip: Risotto is usually made with white short-grain Arborio rice, but brown rice works well, too. Try to find short- or medium-grain brown rice, but in a pinch, you can use long-grain rice.

Spring Quinoa Salad with Apple Cider Dressing

Prep time: 20 min • **Cook time:** 1 hour • **Yield:** 4 servings

Ingredients	Directions
1 cup quinoa	*1* Wash the quinoa and drain.
2 cups water	
1 cup corn kernels	*2* In a large saucepan, bring the water and sea salt to a boil. Add the quinoa and bring the water back to a boil. Cover the pan, and reduce the heat to low so that the contents simmer 25 to 30 minutes, or until all the liquid has been absorbed. Remove the pan from the heat and allow the quinoa to cool.
1 cup chopped walnuts	
1 cup chopped cucumber	
1 apple, peeled and chopped	
2 tablespoons fresh cilantro, chopped	*3* In a small saucepan, bring about ½ inch of water to a boil. Add the corn and cook 2 to 3 minutes, until it's tender. Allow the corn to cool.
2 tablespoons fresh Thai basil, chopped	
2 tablespoons fresh parsley, chopped	*4* Transfer the quinoa to a large mixing bowl and add the walnuts, cucumber, apple, cilantro, basil, parsley, and raisins (if desired). Stir.
½ cup golden raisins (optional)	
Apple Cider Dressing (see the following recipe)	*5* Drizzle the Apple Cider Dressing over the salad and stir it in. Season the salad with the sea salt. Allow the salad to sit for 20 to 30 minutes to allow the flavors to develop before serving.
Pinch of sea salt	

Apple Cider Dressing

¼ cup extra-virgin olive oil	In a small bowl, combine all the ingredients.
¼ cup apple cider vinegar	
Salt and pepper, to taste	

Per serving: Calories 543 (From Fat 321); Fat 36g (Saturated 3g); Cholesterol 0mg; Sodium 309mg; Carbohydrate 43g (Dietary Fiber 15g); Protein 16g.

Cuban Rice and Corn with Black Beans

Prep time: 5 min • **Cook time:** 20 min • **Yield:** 4 servings

Ingredients	Directions
1 tablespoon sesame oil	*1* In a large saucepan, heat the oil.
2 cups organic black beans	
2 teaspoons cumin	*2* Add the black beans, cumin, and sea salt, and cook 3 to 4 minutes.
Pinch sea salt	
2 tablespoons finely chopped fresh cilantro	*3* Stir in the cilantro, and cook 1 minute.
	4 Transfer the beans to a serving dish.
2 ears corn (or, if frozen, 1½ cups)	
	5 In a small saucepan, bring ½ inch of water to boil.
4 cups cooked long-grain brown rice or basmati rice	
2 tablespoons cotija or queso blanco cheese	*6* Cut the kernels from the ears of corn and place them in a steamer over the boiling water. Cook over medium heat for 3 to 4 minutes.
	7 Mix the corn with the rice and transfer to a serving bowl.
	8 Serve the beans over the corn and rice and top with the cheese.

Per serving: Calories 406 (From Fat 62); Fat 7g (Saturated 2g); Cholesterol 3mg; Sodium 222mg; Carbohydrate 74g (Dietary Fiber 10g); Protein 14g.

Seafood

Seafood doesn't usually draw casual opinions; most people love it or hate it. If you don't like seafood, try replacing it with chicken or tofu.

Most types of seafood are very healthy as long as they're not deep fried or covered in tartar sauce. Fish and shellfish are full of high-quality protein and other essential nutrients. They support heart health and are lower in fat than beef or pork.

Keep the following tips in mind when buying fish:

- ✔ Be careful about the temperature of the fish you're buying. Buy it frozen, from a refrigerator, or when it's on top of a thick layer of fresh ice. If the refrigerator seems ill functioning or the layer of ice is sparse or melting too quickly, don't buy the fish.

- ✔ Some seafood products have an indicator on the package that shows whether the seafood has been kept at the right temperature. If the product you're looking at has such an indicator, pay attention to it.

- ✔ If you buy frozen fish, follow the thawing instructions. If you thaw it too slowly, dangerous bacteria can form.

- ✔ Smell it! Fish has an odor, but it shouldn't be strong. Fish should smell fresh, not sour or ammonia-like.

- ✔ When buying a whole fish, look for one that has clear (not cloudy) eyes.

- ✔ Whole fish and fish fillet should be firm and should spring back when you press it.

- ✔ The fish should have shiny flesh.

- ✔ If the fish has a milky slime, avoid it.

- ✔ Fish fillets should not have darkness or be dry around the edges.

One recipe in this section contains shrimp. When buying shrimp, look for ones that are translucent and shiny. They should have no odor, or just a very minimal odor.

The following seafood recipes are high in nutrients and flavor, and they're well balanced to keep you satisfied longer.

Seared Salmon with Sautéed Summer Vegetables

Prep time: 10 min • **Cook time:** 15–20 min • **Yield:** 4 servings

Ingredients	Directions
3 cups broccoli florets	**1** Steam the broccoli florets for 3 to 6 minutes; set aside.
1 tablespoon olive oil	
1 carrot, peeled and cut into ¼-inch-thick rounds	**2** In a large skillet, heat the olive oil. Add the carrot and sauté for 1 to 3 minutes. Add the peppers, broccoli, cucumber, and radishes, and sauté for 1 to 3 minutes. Remove and transfer to a bowl; sprinkle with basil and salt.
1 yellow bell pepper, chopped	
1 red bell pepper, chopped	
1 cucumber, peeled, seeded, and cut into 2-inch spears	**3** In a skillet, heat the coconut oil over medium-high heat. Season the salmon with salt and then add it to the skillet, searing each side for about 4 minutes. After 8 minutes, check to make sure the salmon is cooked through. If it isn't, cook for 1 more minute on each side.
1 bunch of radishes (about 5 radishes), quartered and with some of the greens attached	
4 basil leaves, chopped	**4** Serve the salmon on top of the sautéed vegetables.
¼ teaspoon salt	
1 teaspoon coconut oil	
Four 5-ounce salmon fillets	

Per serving: Calories 272 (From Fat 101); Fat 11g (Saturated 3g); Cholesterol 66mg; Sodium 288mg; Carbohydrate 10g (Dietary Fiber 4g); Protein 33g.

Tip: You can serve the veggies in this recipe with any meat dish.

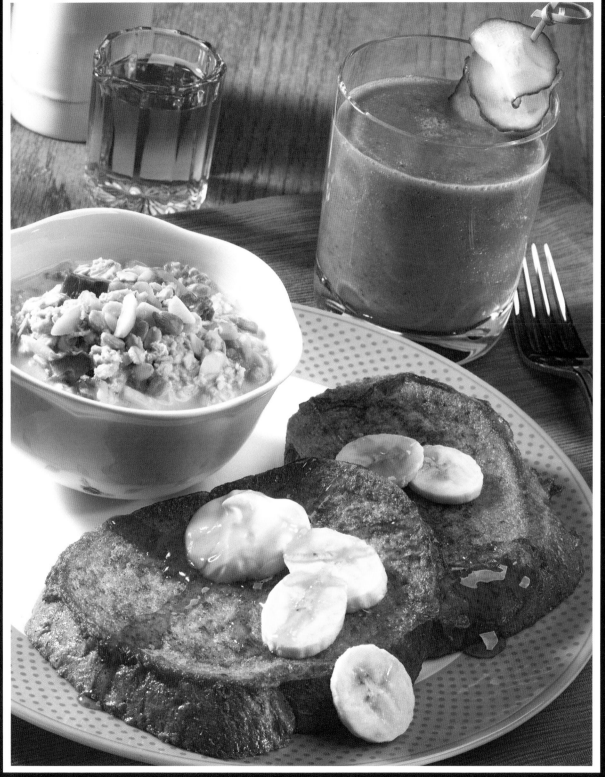

Great Green Smoothies, Fast Morning Muesli, and Fabulous French Toast (all in Chapter 9)

Salmon and New Potato Salad and Carrot Ginger Soup (both in Chapter 10)

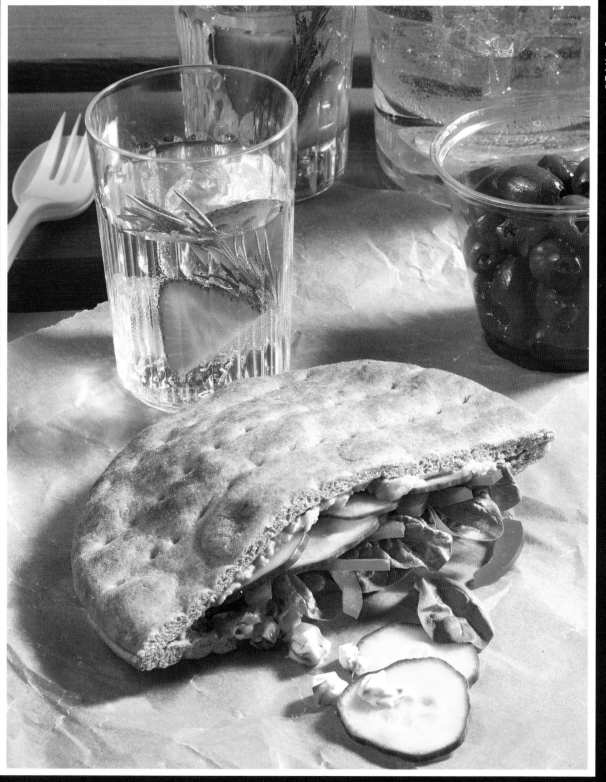

Veggie Pitas (Chapter 10)

Spring Quinoa Salad with Apple Cider Dressing and Seared Salmon with Sautéed Summer Vegetables (both in Chapter 11)

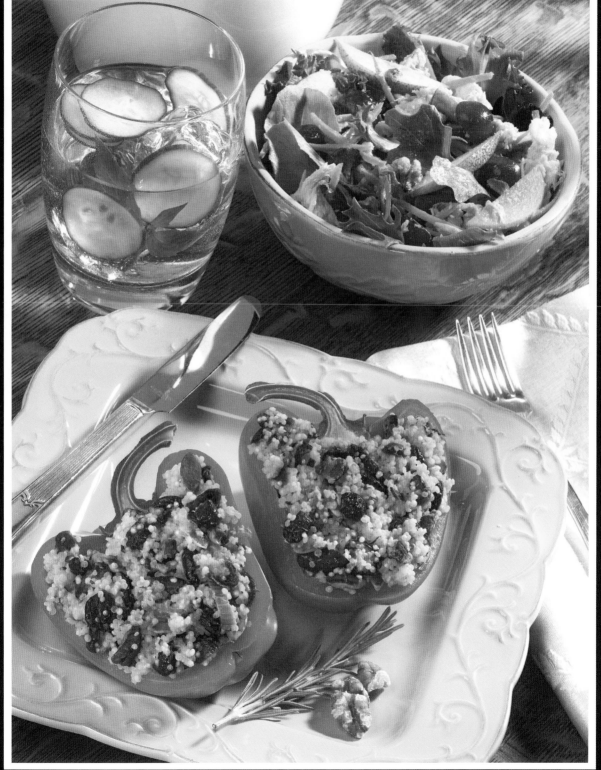

Roast Chicken Salad with Avocado Dressing and Stuffed Sweet Peppers (both in Chapter 11), with Cucumber Water (Chapter 13)

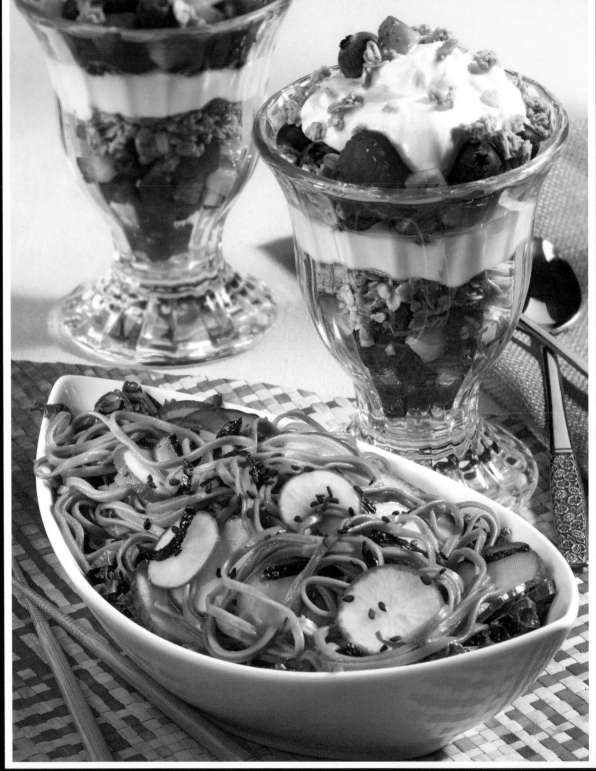

Granola Berry Parfaits and Summer Soba Salad with Sweet Sesame Dressing (both in Chapter 12)

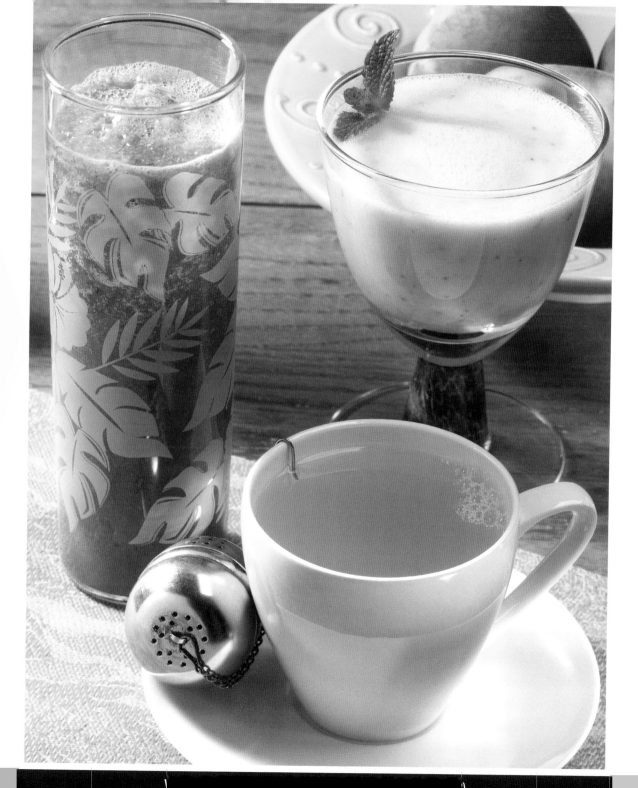

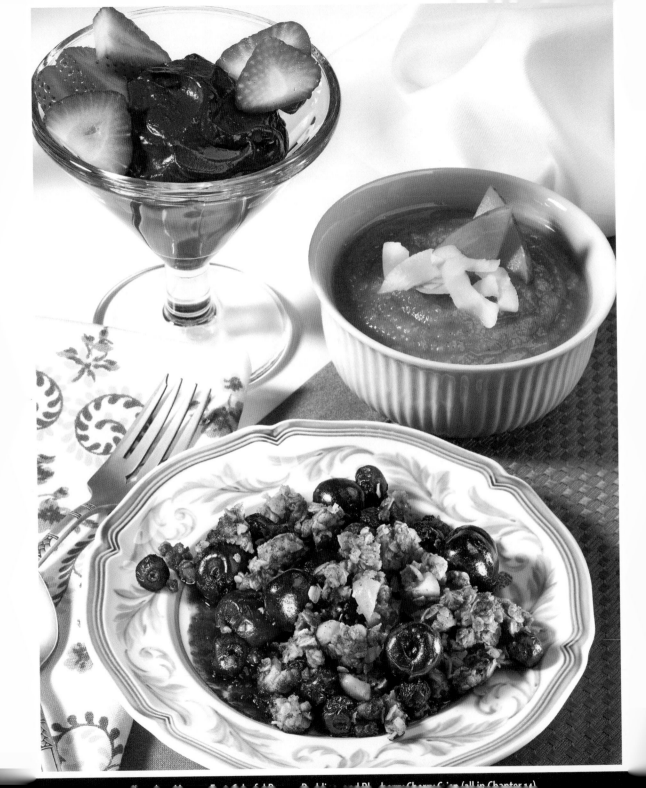

Coconut Panko Shrimp

Prep time: 20 min • **Cook time:** 8 min • **Yield:** 4 servings

Ingredients	Directions
2 pounds large or jumbo shrimp, tail on and deveined	*1* Butterfly the shrimp and set aside in a bowl.
½ cup rough or fine panko flakes	*2* In a bowl, combine the panko flakes and coconut flakes.
One 4-ounce bag sweetened coconut flakes	*3* In a separate bowl, lightly beat the eggs.
4 eggs	*4* Dip the shrimp into the egg and then the panko/coconut mixture and place on a platter.
1 cup coconut oil	*5* When all the shrimp are dressed and ready to go, heat the coconut oil in a skillet over medium-high heat.
	6 Add several shrimp to the skillet, leaving room to turn them when one side is golden brown. Cook for about 2 minutes on each side; remove and drain thoroughly on several layers of paper towel. Repeat for the rest of the shrimp.

Per serving: Calories 557(From Fat 258); Fat 29g (Saturated 22g); Cholesterol 550mg; Sodium 1,800mg; Carbohydrate 25g (Dietary Fiber 3g); Protein 47g.

Tip: To test whether your oil is hot enough for frying, place one coated shrimp into the hot oil to see whether the oil bubbles and sizzles.

Note: It sounds counterintuitive, but when done right, deep frying is not very high in fat. The hot oil cooks the outside without entering the food. This requires a higher cooking temperature (oil should be between 175 and 190 degrees), and the food should be submerged for only a minute or so. Most important, eat a small portion!

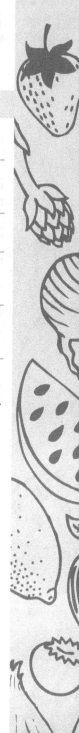

Baked Italian Fish Packets

Prep time: 20 min • **Cook time:** 20–25 min • **Yield:** 4 servings

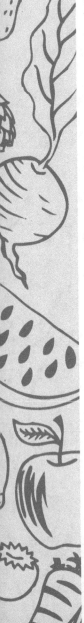

Ingredients	Directions
1 fennel bulb (about 1 pound), cut in half and sliced thin lengthwise	*1* Preheat the oven to 375 degrees. In a medium bowl, combine the fennel, dill, and basil.
½ cup finely chopped fresh dill	*2* In a small bowl, combine the balsamic vinegar, olive oil, mustard, sea salt, and pepper; mix with a whisk until well blended.
2 tablespoons chopped fresh basil	
¼ cup white balsamic vinegar	*3* Cut four 18-x-12-inch sheets of parchment paper and arrange them on your work surface.
¼ cup extra-virgin olive oil	
1 tablespoon Dijon mustard	*4* Place one fish fillet in the center of each sheet of paper. Top each fillet with ¼ of the basil, fennel, and dill mixture, and drizzle each fillet with ¼ of the olive oil mixture.
½ teaspoon sea salt	
⅛ teaspoon pepper	
Four 4- to 6-ounce red snapper fillets	*5* Lift the short sides of the paper and fold the edges together twice to seal them. Then lift and fold the other sides of the paper to seal them together. Be sure to leave some air space in the packet to allow for heat expansion.
	6 Place the fish packets on a cookie sheet. Bake for 20 to 25 minutes, or until the fish flakes when you test it with a fork. (Carefully unwrap one packet and test the fish for doneness.)
	7 Place each packet on a plate. Cut a large X across the top of each packet. Serve immediately, making sure to warn diners to be careful of the steam when they open their packets.

Per serving: Calories 261 (From Fat 134); Fat 15g (Saturated 2g); Cholesterol 40mg; Sodium 460mg; Carbohydrate 8g (Dietary Fiber 2g); Protein 23g.

Note: Baking fish in parchment paper is a wonderful way to keep it moist and tender. The paper also helps hold in all the flavors as the fish cooks, and it's a clean way to cook. You can also wrap the fish in foil and grill it over medium coals for 15 to 20 minutes until the fish flakes when you test it with a fork.

Pasta and Breads

Comfort food, mmm. Now we're talking! Yes, these pasta- and bread-based foods are comforting and heavy on carbs, but they're also well balanced because they include vegetables and protein as well.

Carb controversy

Ever since the 1990s, there has been a controversy over whether carbs are good for us. The answer: Yes.

We need carbohydrates. Our bodies use carbs to make glucose, and glucose is the fuel that gives us energy to, well, stay alive. The body can use glucose immediately, or store it for later when it's needed more. Important stuff.

However, the types and amounts of carbohydrates we eat dictate whether the carbs are a good idea. Balance is key. Unless you're an avid marathon runner, for instance, there's no reason to load up on carbs. If you have a bagel for breakfast, a bowl of spaghetti for lunch, and pizza for dinner, it's time to scale back on the carbs.

Remember: When most people think of the term *carbohydrate*, flour-based items such as pancakes, pasta, and bread come to mind. However, vegetables and fruits are also sources of carbohydrates. Same with milk products and sugar.

Excess carbs can lead to weight gain, but carbs themselves are not a problem. Balance your carb consumption with other types of food and in the rights amounts, and you'll be a-okay.

Vegetable Lasagne with White Sauce

Prep time: 1 hr • **Cook time:** 35 min • **Yield:** 6 servings

Ingredients	Directions
3 tablespoons butter	*1* Preheat the oven to 350 degrees.
4 tablespoons flour	
3 cups lowfat milk	*2* In a medium saucepan, add the butter over low heat. When the butter has melted, slowly stir in the flour with a wooden spoon. Cook for 2 minutes, being careful not to brown the flour. Add the milk to the saucepan and increase the heat to medium. Continue to stir until the milk starts to boil. Reduce the heat and simmer for 1 minute. Remove the saucepan from the heat and whisk the Parmesan cheese into the milk mixture. Add salt and pepper, to taste. Set aside.
½ cup Parmesan cheese	
Salt and pepper, to taste	
1 tablespoon olive oil	
2 cups baby portobello mushrooms, sliced	
1 large carrot, finely sliced	*3* In a skillet, heat the olive oil over medium heat. Add the mushrooms and carrots to the skillet, and sauté until the carrots are tender, about 4 minutes. Set aside.
9 lasagna noodles	
15 ounces lowfat ricotta cheese	
1 egg	*4* Cook the lasagna noodles according to the package instructions and drain.
½ cup Parmesan cheese, grated	*5* Meanwhile, in a medium bowl, combine the ricotta cheese, egg, and grated Parmesan cheese until well mixed.
2 small zucchini, finely sliced	
2 cups baby spinach, roughly chopped	*6* In a 9-x-13-inch baking dish, add ¼ cup of the sauce mixture, spreading the sauce evenly along the bottom of the dish. Place three lasagna noodles on top of the sauce and add 1 cup of ricotta. Layer half the zucchini and half the spinach evenly over the ricotta. Next, layer half the mushroom mixture and 1 cup of the sauce. Add one-third of the mozzarella. Repeat with a noodle layer, ricotta, the remaining vegetables, and another one-third of the mozzarella. Top the second layer with the remaining noodles, sauce, and mozzarella. Cover with foil and bake for 35 minutes.
8 ounces shredded lowfat mozzarella	

Per serving: Calories 480 (From Fat 209); Fat 23g (Saturated 13g); Cholesterol 107mg; Sodium 837mg; Carbohydrate 37g (Dietary Fiber 2g); Protein 34g.

Kale and Carrot Pasta

Prep time: 15 min • **Cook time:** 20 min • **Yield:** 4 servings

Ingredients	*Directions*
One 12-ounce package spaghetti	*1* In a large saucepan, cook the pasta according to the package instructions.
3 tablespoons olive oil	
1 large carrot, finely chopped	*2* Meanwhile, in a large sauté pan, heat 1 tablespoon of the olive oil over medium heat. Add the carrot and bell pepper to the sauté pan and sauté for 4 to 5 minutes, stirring constantly. Add the kale to the pan and sauté an additional 4 minutes.
1 large red bell pepper, finely chopped	
1 bunch kale, stems removed, roughly chopped	
2 tablespoons fresh basil, chopped	*3* Drain the pasta and toss with the remaining 2 tablespoons of olive oil.
¼ cup Parmesan cheese, grated	*4* Toss the kale mixture with the pasta. Top with the basil, Parmesan cheese, and salt and pepper.
Salt and pepper, to taste	

Per serving: Calories 515 (From Fat 131); Fat 15g (Saturated 3g); Cholesterol 4mg; Sodium 281mg; Carbohydrate 78g (Dietary Fiber 7g); Protein 19g.

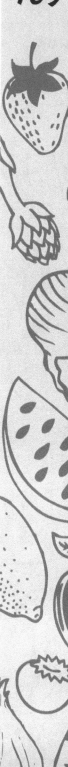

Mushroom, Goat Cheese, and Arugula Flatbread

Prep time: 15 min • **Cook time:** 15 min • **Yield:** 2 servings

Ingredients	Directions
3 tablespoons extra-virgin olive oil	*1* Preheat the oven to 400 degrees.
5 cremini mushrooms, sliced	*2* In a medium sauté pan, heat 1 tablespoon of the olive oil over medium heat. Add the mushrooms to the pan and sauté with the basil and thyme until tender. Set aside.
2 tablespoons fresh basil, chopped	
1 tablespoon fresh thyme, chopped	
1 premade flatbread	*3* On a baking sheet, place the flatbread. Layer with the mushrooms, goat cheese, and arugula. Drizzle the remaining 2 tablespoons of olive oil over the top.
2 tablespoons goat cheese, crumbled	
½ cup arugula	*4* Place the baking sheet in the oven and bake until warm throughout, about 5 minutes.

Per serving: Calories 279 (From Fat 216); Fat 24g (Saturated 4g); Cholesterol 9mg; Sodium 197mg; Carbohydrate 12g (Dietary Fiber 1g); Protein 5g.

Vary It! Cremini mushrooms are a particularly flavorful mushroom and work well in this recipe. However, you can use any other type of mushroom instead if you don't have cremini on hand.

Note: Naan, pita, or pizza crust will also work in place of the flatbread.

Veggie-Based Dishes

Many people grew up with boiled veggies, and that was the problem. Boiling is rarely a great way to cook a vegetable (with the exception of potatoes, and even those can taste better when roasted or baked). Boiling zaps out the flavor and damages some of the nutrients. Perhaps the worst affront, however, is what boiling does to the texture: When a vegetable has been boiled to a limp or slimy pulp, it's hard to bring it back to the land of tastiness, even with the best seasoning.

Instead of boiling, try these methods for cooking veggies:

- ✔ **Steaming:** Bring water to a boil in a pan or pot. Keep it boiling. Put a strainer or a steamer basket above the pan or pot. Put the vegetable in the strainer or steamer basket and cook until the vegetable reaches your desired softness.

- ✔ **Sautéing:** Put a frying pan on a burner and turn the heat to medium or medium-high. When the pan is hot (this will take a minute or two), add a little oil (a tablespoon or so, but it depends on what you're cooking). When the oil is hot, add your ingredients. Stir occasionally. Cook until the vegetable reaches your desired softness.

- ✔ **Roasting:** Heat the oven to 325 degrees. Place the vegetable in a roasting pan or on a baking sheet. Cover with foil if you'd like to increase moisture. Cooking time depends on the vegetable and how much of it you have.

- ✔ **Broiling:** Broiling is somewhere between baking and grilling. You can broil in your oven or with a broiling machine. To use your oven, set it on the broil setting. Place your vegetable on a baking sheet or in a roasting pan. Covering the food is optional.

Or just eat your veggies raw!

Before you throw in the towel on vegetables, make sure you've tried vegetables that are prepared well. The recipes in this section make vegetables the main star — and none of them includes boiling the heck out those poor plants!

Spaghetti Squash

Prep time: 10 min • **Cook time:** 45 min • **Yield:** 4 servings

Ingredients	Directions
One 2-pound spaghetti squash	**1** Preheat the oven to 375 degrees.
1 tablespoon olive oil	**2** Using a sharp knife, cut the squash in half lengthwise. Scoop out the seeds and discard.
¼ cup Parmesan cheese	
2 tablespoons fresh Italian parsley, chopped	**3** On a greased baking dish filled with ½ inch of water, place the squash halves cut side down. Bake until tender, 30 to 45 minutes.
1 teaspoon fresh thyme, minced	
1 teaspoon fresh oregano, minced	**4** When the squash is cool enough to handle, transfer it to a cutting board and use a fork to scrape out the flesh into noodle-like strands. Scoop out the entire contents, all the way to the skin.
Salt and pepper, to taste	
	5 In a large serving bowl, place the squash, olive oil, ⅛ cup of the Parmesan cheese, parsley, thyme, oregano, and salt and pepper. Stir gently to mix well. Top with the remaining cheese.

Per serving: Calories 105 (From Fat 48); Fat 5g (Saturated 2g); Cholesterol 4mg; Sodium 258mg; Carbohydrate 13g (Dietary Fiber 3g); Protein 3g.

Fennel-Stuffed Acorn Squash

Prep time: 20 min • **Cook time:** 1 hr • **Yield:** 4 servings

Ingredients	Directions
2 medium acorn squash, halved and seeded	*1* Preheat the oven to 400 degrees.
1 tablespoon butter	*2* In a large baking dish, place the squash halves flesh side down and bake for 45 minutes.
1 large fennel bulb, trimmed and thinly sliced (see Figure 11-1)	*3* Meanwhile, in a large sauté pan, melt the butter on medium heat. Add the fennel, mushrooms, and thyme to the pan; sauté until the ingredients are tender.
10 ounces baby portobello mushrooms, diced	
1 tablespoon fresh thyme, chopped	*4* Add the cooked quinoa or rice to the pan and mix well with the fennel and mushrooms. Remove from the heat.
2 cups quinoa or brown rice, cooked	
½ cup grated Parmesan cheese	*5* Remove the squash from the oven and turn each half over. Stuff the squash with the ingredients from the sauté pan. Top with the Parmesan, sunflower seeds, and salt and pepper.
¼ cup sunflower seeds	
Salt and pepper, to taste	*6* Return the squash to the oven for another 5 minutes or until the cheese starts to brown.

Per serving: Calories 344 (From Fat 104); Fat 12g (Saturated 4g); Cholesterol 16mg; Sodium 355mg; Carbohydrate 51g (Dietary Fiber 9g); Protein 15g.

HOW TO SLICE A FENNEL BULB

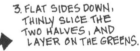
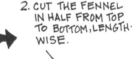
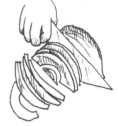
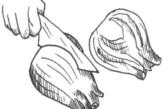
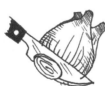

1. CUT A THIN SLICE OFF THE BOTTOM OF THE FENNE BULB TO REMOVE THE ROOT END.

2. CUT THE FENNEL IN HALF FROM TOP TO BOTTOM, LENGTHWISE.

3. FLAT SIDES DOWN, THINLY SLICE THE TWO HALVES, AND LAYER ON THE GREENS.

Figure 11-1: Slicing fennel.

Illustration by Elizabeth Kurtzman

Stuffed Sweet Peppers

Prep time: 15 min • **Cook time:** 45 min • **Yield:** 4 servings

Ingredients	Directions
1 tablespoon olive oil	**1** Preheat the oven to 350 degrees.
2 stalks celery, chopped	**2** In a medium saucepan, heat the oil over medium heat. Add the celery to the pan and sauté until tender. Add the thyme, rosemary, parsley, and salt and pepper, and cook an additional 1 minute.
½ teaspoon dried thyme	
½ teaspoon dried rosemary	
2 tablespoons fresh Italian parsley, chopped	
Salt and pepper, to taste	**3** Stir the quinoa into the celery and add the broth. Cover and bring to a boil. Reduce the heat and simmer for 15 to 20 minutes, until the quinoa is tender.
¾ cup quinoa	
1½ cups low-sodium chicken broth	**4** Stir the cranberries, goat cheese, pumpkin seeds, and pecans into the quinoa.
½ cup dried cranberries	
¼ cup goat cheese, crumbled	**5** Slice a sliver off the bottom of each of the bell peppers so they stay stable in the pan.
2 tablespoons pumpkin seeds, shelled	
2 tablespoons pecans, chopped	**6** In a baking dish, place each halved pepper and fill each pepper with the quinoa mixture.
4 large red bell peppers, seeds removed and halved lengthwise	**7** Cover the peppers with parchment paper and bake for 25 minutes.

Per serving: Calories 341 (From Fat 115); Fat 13g (Saturated 2g); Cholesterol 9mg; Sodium 254mg; Carbohydrate 46g (Dietary Fiber 14g); Protein 11g.

Brown Rice, Vegetable, and Tofu Stir-Fry with Sliced Almonds

Prep time: 10 min • **Cook time:** 15 min • **Yield:** 4 servings

Ingredients	Directions
1 tablespoon extra-virgin olive oil	*1* In a large wok or skillet, heat the olive oil until it's very hot but not smoking.
4 medium carrots, julienned	
1 cup chopped fresh shitake mushrooms	*2* Add the carrots, mushrooms, celery, ginger, basil, and sea salt, and stir-fry over medium-high heat for 3 minutes.
2 stalks celery, cut into slices	
1 tablespoon minced fresh ginger	*3* Add the zucchini and tofu, and cook for 2 minutes.
2 tablespoons fresh chopped Thai basil	*4* Add the greens and stir-fry until they're just wilted (adding a little water if necessary).
Pinch of sea salt	
2 small zucchini, julienned	*5* Stir the almonds into the mixture.
1 pound firm tofu, cut into ½-inch cubes	*6* In a small bowl, mix the tamari with the water and pour over the stir-fried vegetables. Cook for another 2 to 3 minutes.
1 cup finely chopped leafy greens, such as kale or bok choy	
Almond slices, to taste	*7* Transfer the vegetables to a serving dish and serve with the rice.
3 tablespoons tamari	
⅓ cup water	
2 cups cooked brown rice	

Per serving: Calories 306 (From Fat 92); Fat 10g (Saturated 1g); Cholesterol 0mg; Sodium 923mg; Carbohydrate 39g (Dietary Fiber 7g); Protein 17g.

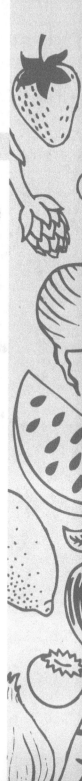

Meats

Acid reflux is a pain, yes? It makes you have to modify your diet and your habits. Annoying! One of those modifications is to steer clear of red meat, or to have only small, infrequent amounts. However, you can still eat meat. The acid reflux diet doesn't require you to be a vegetarian. The seafood recipes earlier in this chapter are great alternatives to vegetarian recipes, and the recipes in this section are great options, too.

Feel free to substitute the meats in this section for any other type of meat, as long as it isn't beef or very high in fat. You can also use vegetarian substitutions such as tofu, tempeh, seitan, or prepared mock-meat substitutes such as "chicken" patties from the frozen section of your local grocery store. There are plenty of great vegetarian options.

Meat can be part of a healthy dinner, as long as you don't have too much of it too often. Americans and people in other industrialized nations tend to eat much more meat than they need to. Too much meat isn't good for your health, because meat is often high in fat. Plus, excess protein is taxing on the kidneys.

Choose lean cuts of meat. And when you do have high-fat meats (hey, everything in moderation, right?), keep the quantities small.

Be sure to store meat at safe temperatures — it should be stored in the refrigerator between 32 and 40 degrees. You can also freeze meat, but to defrost it, put it in the refrigerator instead of out on the countertop. Finally, follow these tips to severely cut your chances of getting sick from meat:

- Wash your hands after touching raw meat.
- Use one cutting board for produce and one for meat, poultry, seafood, and eggs.
- Disinfect countertops after you've prepared raw meat on them. Try to keep the raw meat on a cutting board. Even if you use a cutting board, clean the surrounding areas well.
- Don't allow raw meat to drip in the refrigerator.

Turkey, Fennel, and Apple Couscous

Prep time: 15 min • **Cook time:** 40 min • **Yield:** 4 servings

Ingredients	Directions
2 cups Israeli couscous	**1** In a large pot, cook the couscous according to the package instructions. Drain, return to the pot, and cover.
¼ pound ground turkey	
3 tablespoons olive oil	
1 cup fennel, thinly sliced	**2** Meanwhile, in a large sauté pan, brown the ground turkey. Remove from the pan and set aside.
1 Granny Smith apple, peeled, cored, and thinly sliced	**3** In the same large sauté pan, heat 1 tablespoon of the olive oil over medium-low heat. Add the fennel and apple. Cover and cook, stirring occasionally until the ingredients are tender, about 10 minutes.
¼ cup apple cider	
6 cups baby spinach	
1 teaspoon fresh sage, finely chopped	**4** Uncover and continue to cook, stirring frequently, until the fennel and apple are lightly browned, about 20 minutes.
2 teaspoons fresh thyme, finely chopped	
Salt and pepper, to taste	**5** Add the apple cider to the pan and scrape the bottom to remove any browning.
	6 Add the spinach to the pan, cover, and cook for 2 minutes until wilted.
	7 In a large bowl, combine the couscous, turkey, apple mixture, the remaining 2 tablespoons of olive oil, sage, thyme, and salt and pepper.

Per serving: Calories 434 (From Fat 109); Fat 12g (Saturated 2g); Cholesterol 19mg; Sodium 232mg; Carbohydrate 66g (Dietary Fiber 6g); Protein 14g.

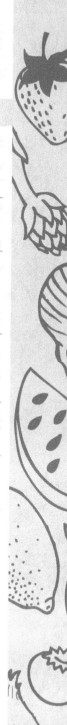

Roasted Pork Tenderloin and Veggies

Prep time: 15 min • **Cook time:** 45–55 min, plus standing time • **Yield:** 8 servings

Ingredients	Directions
3 tablespoons Dijon mustard 3 tablespoons pure maple syrup 1 teaspoon fresh thyme, finely chopped 1 teaspoon dried marjoram ½ teaspoon sea salt ⅛ teaspoon pepper Two 1-pound pork tenderloins 2 large sweet potatoes, peeled and cubed 4 large carrots, cut into 1-inch chunks 2 large parsnips, peeled and cubed 2 cups Brussels sprouts, ends trimmed 2 tablespoons extra-virgin olive oil	*1* Preheat the oven to 375 degrees. In a small bowl, combine the mustard, maple syrup, thyme, marjoram, sea salt, and pepper; mix well. Rub this mixture over the pork tenderloins and set them aside. *2* In a large roasting pan, combine the sweet potatoes, carrots, parsnips, and Brussels sprouts. Drizzle the vegetables with the olive oil and toss to coat evenly. Place the pork tenderloins on top of the vegetables in the pan. *3* Roast the meat and vegetables for 45 to 55 minutes, stirring the vegetables once, until the tenderloin reaches an internal temperature of 155 degrees. Cover and let stand for 5 minutes. Slice the pork tenderloin, and serve it with the vegetables.

Per serving: Calories 264 (From Fat 59); Fat 7g (Saturated 1g); Cholesterol 60mg; Sodium 378mg; Carbohydrate 28g (Dietary Fiber 5g); Protein 24g.

Tip: If your pork tenderloin has one end that's smaller and thinner than the rest of the tenderloin, tuck it under slightly and tie it with kitchen twine so that the whole tenderloin roasts evenly.

Vary It! You can also make this recipe with turkey tenderloin. Just cook the meat until it reaches an internal temperature of 165 degrees.

Roast Chicken Salad with Avocado Dressing

Prep time: 20 min • **Yield:** 2 servings

Ingredients	Directions
4 cups mixed greens	***1*** In a large salad bowl, combine the greens, chicken, and carrot.
1 cup roasted chicken, shredded	
1 small carrot, grated	***2*** Add 2 tablespoons of the Avocado Dressing to the bowl and mix well.
Avocado Dressing (see the following recipe)	
1 small pear, sliced	***3*** Add the pear, grapes, and walnuts to the bowl and toss lightly.
15 red grapes, seeds removed and halved	
10 walnuts, broken into pieces	

Avocado Dressing

1 tablespoon avocado	Place the ingredients in a food processor and blend until smooth.
2 teaspoons extra-virgin olive oil	
½ teaspoon vinegar	
½ teaspoon honey	
Salt and pepper, to taste	

Per serving: Calories 352 (From Fat 153); Fat 17g (Saturated 3g); Cholesterol 62mg; Sodium 440mg; Carbohydrate 27g (Dietary Fiber 6g); Protein 15g.

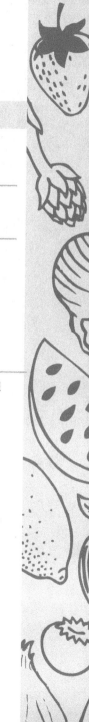

Chapter 12

Appetizers and Snacks

In This Chapter

▶ Making tasty appetizers

▶ Preparing delicious snacks

Appetizers and snacks get blamed for unnecessary calorie consumption, but they can actually be part of a healthy diet, an ideal weight, and a friendly menu for acid reflux sufferers. The appetizers and snacks in this chapter don't have trigger ingredients, but they do have flavor! They're also easy to make because they have few ingredients and few steps. Who says good health has to be difficult?

Appealing Appetizers

The appetizers in this section can be paired with just about any meal. All are healthy and most make vegetables the main star.

All these recipes are good as starters (which is why they're in this section), and you can make them more formal if you're having a fancy dinner. For example, run the Millet Mashed "Potatoes" through a pastry tube to class them up on the plate or in the bowl, sprinkle parsley over the Carrot Fries, or add roasted nuts to one of the dishes. Gourmet in an instant!

If you're not the "courses" type, these appetizers can combine into a great meal, in triplets or pairs. For example, have the Carrot Fries with the Green Chicken Egg Bake and the Sautéed Swiss Chard. Another great combo: the Green Chicken Egg Bake with the Carrot Fries and the Millet Mashed "Potatoes."

Carrot Fries

Prep time: 10 min • **Cook time:** 30 min • **Yield:** 4 servings

Ingredients	Directions
1½ pounds carrots, scrubbed and cut into sticks	*1* Preheat the oven to 425 degrees.
1 tablespoons olive oil	*2* In a mixing bowl, place all the ingredients and mix until evenly coated.
1 tablespoon fresh rosemary, finely chopped	
Salt and pepper, to taste	*3* On a greased baking pan, arrange the carrots in a single layer.
	4 Transfer to the oven and bake until the carrots are tender and lightly browned, about 30 minutes.
	5 Enjoy immediately.

Per serving: Calories 126 (From Fat 60); Fat 7g (Saturated 1g); Cholesterol 0mg; Sodium 277mg; Carbohydrate 15g (Dietary Fiber 4g); Protein 2g.

Vary It! Carrot fries are a healthier version of french fries, and they taste great! If you get tired of them, though, you can substitute the carrots with sweet potatoes. The texture of sweet potatoes is more like a french fry than a carrot fry is, and like carrot fries, sweet potato fries are very healthy — sweet potatoes are high in fiber, potassium, calcium, and vitamins A and C.

Note: By the way, the term *sweet potato* is often used interchangeably with *yam,* but they're different vegetables. Yams are larger and more starchy than a sweet potato. You can make fries out of yams, too, but they may not be as tasty as carrot fries or sweet potato fries.

Sautéed Swiss Chard

Prep time: 5 min • **Cook time:** 10 min • **Yield:** 2 servings

Ingredients	Directions
2 tablespoons pine nuts	*1* In a skillet, dry-toast the pine nuts over low heat until they just start to brown and become fragrant, about 4 minutes. ***Note:*** Pine nuts burn very easily. At first you won't see any difference in color and may think the pine nuts aren't cooking, and then suddenly, they may burn. Watch them carefully and stir every couple minutes. When done, remove from the pan and set aside to cool.
1 tablespoon olive oil	
1 bunch Swiss chard, stems trimmed, leaves chopped	
2 tablespoons golden raisins	
⅛ teaspoon thyme	
Salt and pepper, to taste	*2* Add the olive oil to the pan, and heat for 30 seconds.
Parmesan cheese, grated, for garnish	*3* Add the Swiss chard, raisins, and thyme to the pan, and sauté until the Swiss chard is tender, about 5 minutes.
	4 Add the salt and pepper.
	5 Just before serving, add the cheese and pine nuts.

Per serving: Calories 164 (From Fat 113); Fat 13g (Saturated 1g); Cholesterol 0mg; Sodium 447mg; Carbohydrate 12g (Dietary Fiber 2g); Protein 3g.

Vary It! Not a fan of Swiss chard? You can substitute fresh spinach or kale. Both are super healthy and will work just as well as Swiss chard in this recipe.

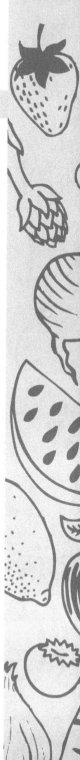

Green Chicken Egg Bake

Prep time: 15 min • **Cook time:** 35 min • **Yield:** 1 serving

Ingredients	Directions
1 teaspoon olive oil or peanut oil	*1* Preheat the oven to 400 degrees. Grease a loaf pan and set aside.
1 stalk celery, diced	
4 ounces chicken breast meat, diced	*2* In a skillet, heat the oil over medium heat. Add the celery and cook for 1 to 2 minutes.
⅛ teaspoon salt	*3* Season the chicken with salt and pepper and add it to the skillet with about ¼ cup of the water. Continue stirring until the chicken is cooked; remove from the heat.
⅛ teaspoon pepper	
⅜ cup water	
2 eggs	*4* In a separate bowl, whisk or beat the eggs and the remaining ⅛ cup of the water with a fork. Add the spinach and any optional ingredients (if desired).
1 cup spinach	
¼ cup cheese, peppers, bacon, or other leftovers (optional)	*5* Place the chicken/celery mixture in the bottom of the loaf pan and cover with the egg/spinach mixture. Bake for about 20 minutes or until a knife comes out clean, meaning the egg is cooked.

Per serving: Calories 388 (From Fat 162); Fat 18g (Saturated 5g); Cholesterol 468mg; Sodium 613mg; Carbohydrate 6g (Dietary Fiber 2g); Protein 48g.

Vary It! Sprinkle the cheese on top of the dish as it bakes instead of mixing it in with the eggs.

Tip: If the spinach is poking out and getting burned, you can add more eggs to cover everything up.

Summer Soba Salad with Sweet Sesame Dressing

Prep time: 10 min • **Cook time:** 30 min • **Yield:** 4 servings

Ingredients	Directions
1 medium cucumber, finely sliced	*1* In a medium bowl, place the cucumber, radishes, and wakame; add the salt, and let sit for about 15 minutes.
6 radishes, finely sliced	
½ cup dry wakame, finely sliced	*2* Cook the noodles according to the package directions, rinse under cool water, and drain.
½ teaspoon sea salt	
One 12-ounce package soba noodles	*3* Pour the excess liquid off the vegetables and add the noodles.
Sweet Sesame Dressing (see the following recipe)	*4* Pour the Sweet Sesame Dressing over the salad and mix gently. Let sit for 15 minutes.
½ cup water	
5 kale leaves, stalk removed and roughly chopped	*5* In a shallow pan, boil the water. Add the kale and cook over a high heat for 1 to 2 minutes to blanch the leaves.
1 tablespoon crushed toasted black sesame seeds, for garnish	*6* Serve on a bed of blanched kale garnished with the sesame seeds.

Sweet Sesame Dressing

3 tablespoons shoyu	*1* In a small bowl, place all the ingredients and mix together.
2 tablespoons mirin	
2 tablespoons honey	
1 tablespoon toasted sesame oil	
6 tablespoons brown rice vinegar	

Per serving: Calories 452 (From Fat 44); Fat 5g (Saturated 1g); Cholesterol 0mg; Sodium 1,379mg; Carbohydrate 87g (Dietary Fiber 2g); Protein 20g.

Millet Mashed "Potatoes"

Prep time: 5 min • **Cook time:** 40 min • **Yield:** 4 servings

Ingredients	Directions
1 cup millet	**1** In a medium skillet, lightly roast the millet by stirring over medium-low heat until it smells toasty, about 5 to 8 minutes.
3 cups water	
1 cup cauliflower florets	
¼ teaspoon salt	**2** In a large saucepan, bring the water to a boil over high heat, and add the millet, cauliflower, and salt.
1 teaspoon tamari	
Sprig of parsley, for garnish	**3** Cover the pan, reduce the heat to low, and simmer for 25 minutes.
	4 Add the tamari and cook for an additional 5 minutes.
	5 Using a potato masher or a hand blender, mash the millet and cauliflower, adding water if necessary.
	6 Place in a serving bowl and garnish with the parsley.

Per serving: Calories 454 (From Fat 35); Fat 4g (Saturated 1g); Cholesterol 0mg; Sodium 233mg; Carbohydrate 90g (Dietary Fiber 6g); Protein 14g.

Super Snacks

Some nutritionists say snacking between meals is bad — they claim that snacking can lead to weight gain. And it can. But if you choose the right snacks in the right quantities and balance them with the right meals in the right quantities, you shouldn't gain weight.

In fact, keeping your meals small and snacking in between is a great route for people who suffer from acid reflux. The digestive system can handle food in small, frequent quantities better than it can handle a glutton fest. Plus, snacking keeps blood sugar steady, and stable blood sugar is a pillar of good health. Here's why:

- **Steady blood sugar keeps you from getting dizzy.** Ever felt like you were going to pass out when you've been hungry too long? Chances are, your blood sugar was too low.

- **Steady blood sugar helps prevent diabetes.** When blood sugar is too high for too long a period of time (weeks, months, or years), a person can become pre-diabetic, and eventually, diabetic.

- **Steady blood sugar helps prevent diabetes-related conditions.** People who have diabetes have an increased risk of stroke, heart disease, kidney problems, vision problems, and more. Diabetes is serious business.

To keep blood sugar stable, don't go more than four hours without eating (except for when you're sleeping, of course). Some people need to eat every hour or two to keep their blood sugar stable. That's okay. Try to avoid high-sugar snacks and beverages such as cookies and soda. Consume protein and fiber — they get digested more slowly than treats, and that means the sugar in them hits the blood stream more slowly. Junk food gets broken down too quickly, and when we break foods down very quickly (such as a tablespoon of white sugar) that food hits the blood stream too fast and can spike blood sugar. The snacks in this chapter are a great way to keep you satisfied between meals, and to keep that all-important blood sugar happy. And, of course, they're acid reflux friendly!

Kale Chips

Prep time: 10 min • **Cook time:** 15 min • **Yield:** 2 servings

Ingredients	Directions
1 bunch kale, stems removed, torn into 2-inch pieces (about 3 to 4 cups total)	*1* Preheat the oven to 425 degrees.
1 tablespoons olive oil	*2* In a mixing bowl, place all the ingredients, and mix until the kale is evenly coated.
Salt and pepper, to taste	*3* On a greased baking pan, arrange the kale in a single layer.
	4 Transfer to the oven and bake until the kale is crispy and lightly browned, about 10 to 15 minutes.
	5 Enjoy immediately.

Per serving: Calories 169 (From Fat 128); Fat 14g (Saturated 2g); Cholesterol 0mg; Sodium 329mg; Carbohydrate 9g (Dietary Fiber 2g); Protein 4g.

Vary It! This recipe is about as easy as it gets, and it's just as easy if you substitute the kale with spinach or Swiss chard. Try making this recipe the same day you make the Sautéed Swiss Chard (earlier in this chapter), and use whatever green you use for one recipe in the other recipe, too.

Apple with Almond Butter

Prep time: 15 min • **Yield:** 2 servings

Ingredients	Directions
1 apple, cored and cut into slices	*1* Dip the apple slices into the almond butter.
2 tablespoons almond butter	*2* Enjoy!

Per serving: Calories 146 (From Fat 81); Fat 9g (Saturated 1g); Cholesterol 0mg; Sodium 37mg; Carbohydrate 16g (Dietary Fiber 4g); Protein 4g.

Make your own almond butter

Want to make your own almond butter? It's easy! In a food processor, combine the following ingredients:

- 15 ounces roasted almonds (raw will work, too, but they may not taste as good)

- 1 teaspoon salt

- 1 or 2 teaspoons honey (optional)

- 2 or 3 tablespoons peanut oil or vegetable oil (optional)

Blend for one minute (or more if you like your almond butter smooth). Store in an airtight container in the refrigerator to give the almond butter its longest shelf life (about two months). It will be harder to spread when cold, so leave it out for an hour or two at room temperature if you like.

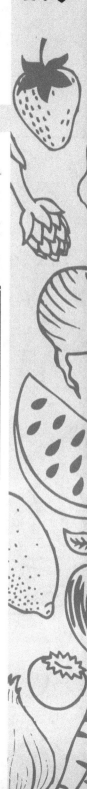

Tuna Salad, Hold the Mayo

Prep time: 5 min • **Cook time:** 8 min • **Yield:** 1 serving

Ingredients	Directions
1 hardboiled egg, diced small	**1** In a small bowl, place the egg and avocado.
¼ avocado	
2 to 3 tablespoons plain yogurt	**2** Add the yogurt. *Note:* You may need only 2 tablespoons if your yogurt of choice isn't very thick.
One 5-ounce can tuna in water, drained	
⅛ teaspoon salt, or to taste	**3** Add the tuna, salt, and pepper, and mash together.
⅛ teaspoon pepper, or to taste	

Per serving: Calories 326 (From Fat 133); Fat 15g (Saturated 3g); Cholesterol 247mg; Sodium 908mg; Carbohydrate 6g (Dietary Fiber 1g); Protein 42g.

Vary It! You can add celery, apples, or different seasonings to jazz up this tuna salad even more.

Easy Edamame Ecstasy

Cook time: 8 minutes • **Yield:** 4 servings

Ingredients	Directions
One 16-ounce package frozen edamame	*1* In a medium saucepan, cook the edamame according to the package directions.
2 teaspoons sea salt, or to taste	*2* Drain the edamame and place it in a serving bowl.
	3 Sprinkle the sea salt over the edamame, making sure that all the pods get a few granules, and serve.

Per serving: Calories 605 (From Fat 163); Fat 18g (Saturated 0g); Cholesterol 0mg; Sodium 763mg; Carbohydrate 54g (Dietary Fiber 24g); Protein 48g.

Balancing choices

Often, the more food choices we have, the more we eat. And as you know, if you eat meals that are too big, all that food puts pressure on the lower esophageal sphincter (LES), which can increase acid reflux. If you're having a meal that includes appetizers, simply eat less of the main meal than you would eat if you didn't have an appetizer. If you have several snacks in a day, eat smaller meals.

Maintaining a healthy weight is an important part of acid reflux prevention, and a big part of healthy weight is paying attention to calories in versus calories out. People tend to complicate weight loss, but for the most part (with

the exception of thyroid problems and other rare disorders), anyone can lose weight if she burns more calories than she consumes. What foods those calories come from is less important for weight loss than the amount of calories consumed. For acid reflux, however, the type of food is important, too — simply reducing calories isn't usually enough to keep acid reflux away.

The healthy appetizer recipes in this chapter can all be enjoyed with an entrée, and the snacks can complement meals. Balance the quantities, and you'll be fine.

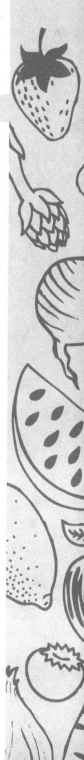

Granola Berry Parfaits

Prep time: 15 min • **Yield:** 4 servings

Ingredients	Directions
1 cup fresh raspberries 1 cup fresh blueberries	**1** In a bowl, place the raspberries, blueberries, and strawberries, and toss them gently.
½ cup chopped fresh strawberries 2 cups crushed granola	**2** In each of four parfait glasses, layer the berry mixture, granola, and yogurt; repeat the layers two or three times, depending on the size of the glasses.
1½ cups lowfat Greek or regular yogurt	**3** Serve immediately.

Per serving: Calories 285 (From Fat 40); Fat 4g (Saturated 1g); Cholesterol 5mg; Sodium 41mg; Carbohydrate 51g (Dietary Fiber 5g); Protein 15g.

Note: When you're shopping for granola, choose one that's lower in fat and sugar.

Tip: Use the freshest and most beautiful berries you can find in the market. Or thaw some organic frozen berries and use them instead. If you don't like the texture of frozen berries, just puree them before using them in this recipe.

Tip: If you're not ready to serve these parfaits right after you make them, you can cover and store them for up to 8 hours in the refrigerator. Note that the granola will be a little softer.

Chapter 13

Easing and Pleasing Beverages

In This Chapter

▶ Setting down with a cup of tea

▶ Flavoring your water

▶ Enjoying a healthy fruit drink

*I*f you have acid reflux and you've been paying attention to triggers, you've probably realized that many drinks spur that fiery demon. Soda, beer, wine, booze, mixed drinks, strong fruit juices (especially citrus based), coffee — in other words, all the fun stuff! Amount is also a big issue. For some people, one glass of the aforementioned beverages is okay, but two or more is a problem.

The beverages in this chapter are great because they won't trigger acid reflux, they're refreshing, and they're easy to make. Another benefit: When you find favorites, you'll want to make them often and you'll be motivated to drink them, which will keep you hydrated. The average American is mildly dehydrated most of the time. That's bad news. Even mild dehydration can cause headaches, bad moods, dizziness or confusion, dry mouth, and fatigue.

To keep these symptoms away, drink at least eight glasses (about 8 ounces each) of water a day. Beverages that are heavy on water but have other ingredients are okay, too, as long as they don't have acid reflux triggers. Plenty of tasty options follow.

Tantalizing Teas

Yes, you may miss your coffee. It's hard to replace the comfort and deliciousness of a latte or mocha or even a plain old cup of Joe. But because coffee is a trigger for many people with acid reflux, you may want (or need) to cut down on coffee or cut it out all together. A lovely substitute: tea. Tea isn't as rich as coffee, but the upside is that it's more refreshing.

Some people think tea is too mild. To make the flavors stronger, steep the tea longer and/or add more sweetener. It will also gain more flavor as it sits (after the brewing process).

You can make a big batch of these teas, or just a single serving. You can drink them hot or cold. Finally, each of the teas in this section can be made with caffeine or without. Caffeine is a diuretic, which means it's dehydrating, but a little caffeine shouldn't be a problem unless you have other conditions that are exacerbated by caffeine, such as certain heart problems.

Each of these recipes can be made with a regular tea kettle (or even a simple pot) or an electric tea kettle. You can use tea bags or, for loose-leaf tea, a tea strainer (see Figure 13-1 for strainer options). Each of these options works well — which one you use is just a matter of personal preference.

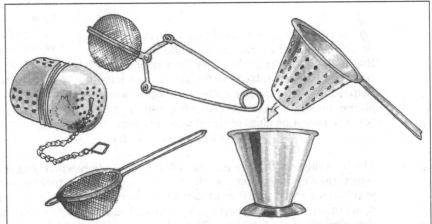

Figure 13-1: Various tea strainers.

Illustration by Elizabeth Kurtzman

"Not for all the tea in China." Guess which country produces the most tea? You got it: China! China alone produces almost 30 percent of the world's supply. That's not a big surprise. India, Vietnam, Iran, Turkey, and Argentina are also big suppliers.

Fresh Ginger Tea

Prep time: 5 min • **Yield:** 1 serving

Ingredients	Directions
One 2-inch piece fresh ginger, peeled and thinly sliced	**1** Steep the ginger in the water for 5 minutes, and serve.
1 cup boiling water	

Per serving: Calories 0 (From Fat 0); Fat 0g (Saturated 0g); Cholesterol 0mg; Sodium 0mg; Carbohydrate 0g (Dietary Fiber 0g); Protein 0g.

Vary It! Some people find tea bland and boring. It can take a little while to get used to the more nuanced flavor of tea, and some people never do. Flavoring your tea can give it that verve you may desire. To incorporate more flavor into this tea, or any tea, steep the tea longer. After it's steeped, add sugar, honey, a few teaspoons of juice, or a splash of milk.

Ginger: Tastes good, feels great

Ginger is a healthy food and is even healthier in its full form than when it's processed into a tea. That's why this recipe uses the fresh variety. Ginger has chemicals that may reduce inflammation. That's great news, because inflammation is the cause of a great many diseases and disorders, from skin problems to irritable bowel syndrome (IBS). Some researchers believe that the chemicals in ginger can soothe the stomach and intestines and may even tell the brain to control nausea. That's why ginger is often used to treat stomach issues, including morning sickness, motion sickness, general upset stomach, colic, gas, diarrhea, and lack of appetite. There is also evidence that ginger can be good for cold and flu symptoms such as congestion.

Ginger can be consumed dried, fresh, or mixed into items like gummies or hard candies. The fresh state is the best, though. When ginger is fresh, more of its nutritional properties are kept in tact than when it goes through the drying process.

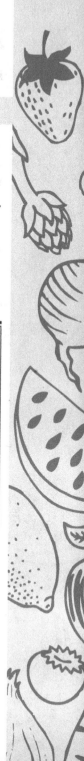

Nettle Iced Tea

Prep time: 10 min • **Yield:** 1 serving

Ingredients	Directions
1 nettle teabag	**1** Steep the teabag and ginger in the water for 10 minutes.
One 2-inch piece fresh ginger, peeled and thinly sliced	
1 cup boiling water	**2** Allow the tea to cool. Then remove the tea bag and ginger from the water.
½ cup crushed ice	
5 to 10 blueberries, for garnish	**3** Pour the tea over the ice, garnish with the blueberries, and serve.

Per serving: Calories 4 (From Fat 0); Fat 0g (Saturated 0g); Cholesterol 0mg; Sodium 0mg; Carbohydrate 1g (Dietary Fiber 0g); Protein 0g.

Nettles 101

So, what are nettles? They don't sound like the most appealing plant ever, and hikers know to stay away from stinging nettle unless they really want a rash in the wilderness. However, the nettle root and part of the above-ground plant may have impressive healing properties when consumed.

Some nutritionists believe that the nettle herb reduces inflammation, is an astringent, and helps with bladder problems. The scientific community isn't conclusive about all the proposed nutrition benefits of nettles, but what you can be confident about is that nettle tea isn't going to exacerbate your acid reflux.

Roasted Barley Tea

Prep time: 3–5 min • **Yield:** 1 serving

Ingredients	Directions
1 roasted barley teabag	*1* Steep the teabag in the water for 3 to 5 minutes and serve. Mix in honey if desired.
1 cup boiling water	
Honey, optional	

Per serving: Calories 0 (From Fat 0); Fat 0g (Saturated 0g); Cholesterol 0mg; Sodium 0mg; Carbohydrate 0g (Dietary Fiber 0g); Protein 0g.

Note: This rich, full-bodied, and soothing after-meal tea is known in Japan as *mugi-cha.* In Japanese, *mugi* means barley. You can buy this tea in commercial Japanese markets, as well as large natural food markets.

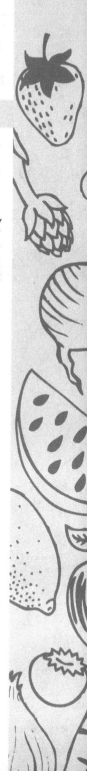

Red Bush Tea (Rooibos Tea)

Prep time: 3–5 min • **Yield:** 1 serving

Ingredients	Directions
1 rooibos teabag	*1* Steep the teabag in the water for 3 to 5 minutes and serve.
1 cup boiling water	

Per serving: Calories 0 (From Fat 0); Fat 0g (Saturated 0g); Cholesterol 0mg; Sodium 0mg; Carbohydrate 0g (Dietary Fiber 0g); Protein 0g.

Note: Popular in South Africa for generations and now consumed in many countries, Rooibos (pronounced *roy*-boss), sometimes called African Red Bush Tea, contains a high level of antioxidants and no caffeine. It has low tannin levels compared to fully oxidized black tea or unoxidized green tea leaves and has a subtle sweet natural taste with a hint of nut flavoring.

Flavored Waters

The best drink for anyone with acid reflux is good old-fashioned water. Ice cold or piping hot, water is the answer. Other drinks have a combination of sugar, acid, carbonation, alcohol, or caffeine that can exacerbate acid reflux, but water is free of all of that. There is absolutely nothing about water that will trigger acid reflux. Drink up!

The only problem with water is that it can get a little boring. A popular way to jazz it up is to add lemon. A few squirts of lemon juice probably won't make your acid reflux act up, but it's a good idea to avoid lemon water anyway. The good news is, there are plenty of other ways to add flavor to your water without using citrus. This section includes "berry good" spa water and cucumber water. Those are refreshing and will soothe troubled throats. Many other ingredients will do the trick as well. Avoid orange, kiwi, cranberry, and pineapple. But try any of the following:

Basil	Blackberries	Cantaloupe
Cherry	Fresh ginger root	Grapes
Honeydew melon	Lavender	Mango
Papaya	Raspberries	Rosemary
Strawberries	Watermelon	

There are dozens of wonderful combinations as well, including the following:

- Blackberry and ginger
- Blackberry and thyme
- Cantaloupe and watermelon
- Papaya and mango
- Strawberry and rosemary
- Watermelon and rosemary

Just juice any of those fruits and herbs and pour a little into your water, or cut pieces of fruit and some herbs and put those in your water. You can leave them there or strain them out. The longer you leave them in the water, the more flavorful the drink will be.

Berry Good Spa Water

Prep time: 15 min • **Yield:** 4 servings

Ingredients	Directions
8 strawberries, halved, fresh or frozen	**1** In a pitcher or beverage dispenser, add the berries to the water.
12 blueberries, fresh or frozen	
8 raspberries, fresh or frozen	**2** Let sit for at least ten minutes in the refrigerator before enjoying. Let the berries sit longer if they're frozen.
4 blackberries, fresh or frozen	
32 ounces filtered water	

Per serving: Calories 16 (From Fat 0); Fat 0g (Saturated 0g); Cholesterol 0mg; Sodium 0mg; Carbohydrate 4g (Dietary Fiber 2g); Protein 0g.

Bottled, filtered, or tap?

Do you ever wonder what's best: bottled water, filtered water, or tap water? Some places have better tap water than others, but overall, it's not going to make a big difference whether you drink bottled water, filtered water, or tap water.

Most bottled water is pretty much the same as tap water anyway. It doesn't hurt to filter your water, though, so if you're worried about the water quality in your area, take the safe route and buy a filter.

Cucumber Water

Prep time: 35 min • **Yield:** 4 servings

Ingredients	Directions
½ cucumber, thinly sliced	*1* In a pitcher, add the cucumber and basil (if desired) to the water.
1 sprig Thai basil (optional)	
32 ounces filtered water	*2* Let sit for at least 30 minutes in the refrigerator before enjoying. Serve at room temperature, refrigerated, or over ice, whichever you prefer.

Per serving: Calories 4 (From Fat 0); Fat 0g (Saturated 0g); Cholesterol 0mg; Sodium 0mg; Carbohydrate 1g (Dietary Fiber 0g); Protein 0g.

Tip: The longer this water sits, the more flavor it will have.

Tip: This recipe makes great ice cubes! Or make ice cubes with fresh juice and serve them in the cucumber water.

Note: Thai basil is an herb native to Southeast Asia. It's a little heartier than regular basil. It can stay in tact in higher cooking temperatures and has a stronger flavor than the type of basil used in Italian cuisine, for instance.

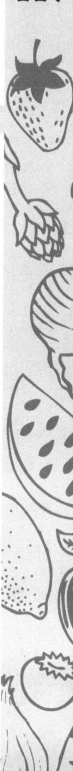

Fruit Drinks

Craving sweetness? What about flavor and freshness? Juice can be the answer. However, people with acid reflux need to be a little more careful with juice than other people have to be:

- ✔ Avoid tomato juice and citrus juices.

- ✔ Avoid juice when it's at full strength, unless you're drinking only a small quantity.

- ✔ Don't drink juice right before you lie down.

- ✔ If you're trying to lose weight, be mindful of the high calorie content in juice. Yet another reason to water it down or go heavy on the ice.

In each of the recipes in this section, and any beverage recipe, fresh juice is always better than bottled. Fruits and vegetables contain enzymes that are killed in the bottling process. When you drink the juice soon after you make it, the enzymes are still alive and can be great for health. Enzymes can help ward off disease and help with the absorption of other nutrients. The fresher the juice, the more enzymes you're getting, and the more vitamins, too.

The easiest and cheapest way to get fresh juice on a regular basis is to buy a juicer. There is a huge price range for juicers, but even if you buy an expensive one (a few hundred dollars) you'll recoup the price within a year if you're a big juice drinker. If you buy a juicer, don't think you need to get one that's top of the line. Even a $40 juicer can do a great job.

A downside to juicers: There's a lot of waste involved with any model, as you'll see by all the pulp even the best juicer spits out. This "waste" material is fantastic for the compost pile, though. You can even just throw it in the garden in a thin layer, and nature will take care of it.

Fresh juice is a little thicker than bottled juice and it separates easily. Give it a good stir, and it will look a lot more appetizing. When people start drinking fresh juice, sometimes they're turned off by the viscous nature and the pulpiness, but if they give it a chance, they're hooked. Bottled apple juice, for instance, can seem tinny and lifeless in comparison.

Note: Each of the recipes in this section will be healthier and taste better with fresh juice, but if you can't get fresh juice or make it, never fear; the recipe will still be good and shouldn't activate your acid reflux.

Hot Apple Ginger Cider

Prep time: 5 min • **Yield:** 1 serving

Ingredients	Directions
One 2-inch piece fresh ginger, peeled and thinly sliced	**1** Steep the ginger in the boiling water for 5 minutes.
4 ounces boiling water	**2** Add the apple cider to the ginger tea and serve hot.
4 ounces apple cider, warmed	

Per serving: Calories 65 (From Fat 0); Fat 0g (Saturated 0g); Cholesterol 0mg; Sodium 13mg; Carbohydrate 16g (Dietary Fiber 0g); Protein 0g.

Making your own apple cider

During the fall, it's pretty easy to find apple cider, but if store-bought cider isn't available, or you'd rather make your own, go for it! You just need 8 medium apples (any variety), water, ¾ cup sugar, 4 tablespoons cinnamon, and 4 tablespoons all-spice. Follow these steps:

1. Peel and quarter the apples.

2. Add the apples to a stock pot and add water over top of the apples. Bring to a boil.

3. Add the sugar to the pot.

4. Put 4 tablespoons of cinnamon and 4 table-spoons of all-spice into a cheese cloth and tie the bundle. Add bundle to the pot.

5. Boil the mixture uncovered for 1 hour.

6. Cover, lower the heat, and simmer for 2 hours.

7. Remove from the heat and let cool completely.

8. Remove the cheese cloth bundle.

9. Mash the apple mixture and send it through a strainer repeatedly until most of the liquid has been removed. That liquid is your cider.

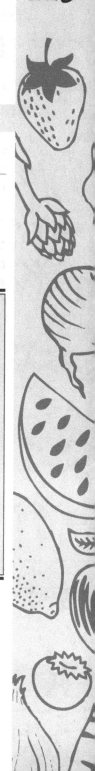

Watermelon Juice

Prep time: 2 min • **Yield:** 4 servings

Ingredients	Directions
½ small watermelon, chilled, cubed	*1* Add the watermelon and basil to a blender.
About 5 basil leaves	*2* Blend until the watermelon is liquefied. Serve.

Per serving: Calories 53 (From Fat 0); Fat 0g (Saturated 0g); Cholesterol 0mg; Sodium 2mg; Carbohydrate 13g (Dietary Fiber 1g); Protein 1g.

Vary It! Any herb will work well with this juice. For example, try rosemary or thyme. Also, if you want the juice to be thinner, clearer, and less pulpy, juice the watermelon instead, and then add water to it.

Peach Kefir

Prep time: 5 min • **Yield:** 1 serving

Ingredients	Directions
6 ounces plain kefir	*1* In a blender, mix all the ingredients until well blended. Serve.
1 peach, halved with pit removed	
2 teaspoons fresh ginger, peeled, chopped	

Per serving: Calories 171 (From Fat 57); Fat 6g (Saturated 0g); Cholesterol 30mg; Sodium 79mg; Carbohydrate 23g (Dietary Fiber 2g); Protein 7g.

Tip: You can use frozen peaches if fresh aren't available. If using frozen peaches, use ½ cup.

What is kefir?

Kefir is a little bit like yogurt. Both are white and made from milk. Both have a tart, tangy taste. Kefir originated in Eastern Europe and contains bacteria from the fermentation process. Not so yummy sounding? Well, yogurt is also fermented, so if you're okay with yogurt, kefir shouldn't be much of a stretch. Yogurt and kefir have different types of bacteria, but the bacteria in both products can be great for digestion.

If kefir isn't your cup of tea, substitute yogurt in this recipe. If you do want to try kefir, you can find it in any health food store and some standard grocery stores.

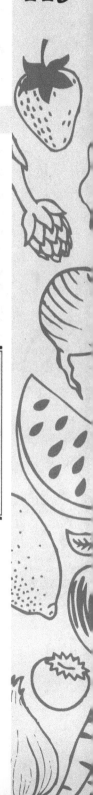

Avocado Smoothies

Prep time: 3 min • **Yield:** 2 servings

Ingredients	*Directions*
12 red grapes	**1** In a blender, mix all the ingredients until smooth. Serve.
1 banana, peeled and halved	
½ avocado, peeled, seed removed	
¾ cup coconut water or plain water	
¼ cup ice or half a frozen banana	

Per serving: Calories 151 (From Fat 53); Fat 6g (Saturated 1g); Cholesterol 0mg; Sodium 7mg; Carbohydrate 26g (Dietary Fiber 3g); Protein 2g.

Chapter 14

Worry-Free Desserts

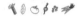
W hen you think of a health-related cookbook, decadent desserts probably don't come to mind. However, rich desserts actually can still be part of your life, even if you have acid reflux. There are many desserts besides the ten in this chapter that you can have as well. For example, fruit (except citrus) is always a good choice. The only dessert to watch out for (besides desserts that are heavy on citrus and/or fat) are those that are heavy on chocolate. Two recipes in this chapter are chocolate based, but they're lower in fat than many chocolate recipes — that's the key. When you have too much fat with too much cocoa, that's when you're in trouble.

The exact ingredients in a recipe aren't the biggest factors for whether a recipe will exacerbate your acid reflux. Instead, watch out for these factors:

✔ **Combination of ingredients:** Does the dessert include citrus and cocoa and a lot of fat? Those are three triggers. You may be able to handle one or two triggers, but probably not three.

✔ **Portion size:** You'd be better off eating a small amount of a citrus-intensive recipe than a huge amount of a dessert that doesn't include acid reflux triggers. Keep your portions small. *Remember:* The human stomach is only about the size of a fist. Yes, it stretches, but even an eighth of a cake can fill the stomach. That's an awful lot of an important body part to take up completely with dessert. The more pressure in the stomach, the more pressure on the lower esophageal sphincter (LES), and that means an increased chance for acid reflux.

✔ **Fat quantity:** High amounts of fat make acid reflux worse. The recipes in this chapter are lower in fat than most dessert recipes, but even these recipes shouldn't be eaten in large quantities.

Puddings and Mousses

Pudding and mousse? The word *yummy* is necessary here. Maybe even *delish*. Well, delish isn't a word. But still.

You may think of puddings and mousses as rich, and rich often means high in fat. As you know, high-fat foods can increase reflux. These recipes, however, are much lower in fat than standard recipes for puddings and mousses. As long as you keep your portions moderate and eat well for your acid reflux the rest of the day, you'll probably tolerate these desserts well.

So, what's moderate? That depends on several factors. For instance, your size and activity level. For the most part, though, we should all follow similar guidelines and those guidelines revolve around the size of our stomachs. Whenever you're dealing with dessert, less is always better than more, at least when it comes to your health. A tablespoon of pudding or mousse is less likely to cause acid reflux than a bowl of it. "But a tablespoon isn't enough!" you say. Well, you're right! How about a champagne glass full? Now you're talking. . . .

Puddings and mousses are creamy, smooth desserts. Some people love that. Others aren't crazy about smooth, one-texture desserts. If you're in the latter category, you can easily make these super-soft desserts more up your alley. How? Sprinkle granola over the top. Another idea: Make a crust, spread the pudding or mousse over the crust, add fruit or granola to that, or spread nut butter over the crust, and you have a dessert that's sophisticated enough to serve to the queen of England, especially if she has acid reflux.

Dreamy Rice Pudding

Prep time: 5 min • **Cook time:** 30 min • **Yield:** 4–6 servings

Ingredients	Directions
1 cup amasake (or rice milk)	*1* In a large saucepan, combine all the ingredients except the vanilla.
½ cup apple juice	
2 cups brown rice	*2* Simmer over medium-low heat for 20 to 30 minutes, stirring often to prevent sticking, until thick and creamy.
3 tablespoons raisins	
3 tablespoons sunflower seeds	
1 teaspoon cinnamon	*3* Stir in the vanilla (if desired), and serve warm or chilled.
1 teaspoon vanilla (optional)	

Per serving: Calories 218 (From Fat 40); Fat 5g (Saturated 1g); Cholesterol 0mg; Sodium 29mg; Carbohydrate 41g (Dietary Fiber 4g); Protein 5g.

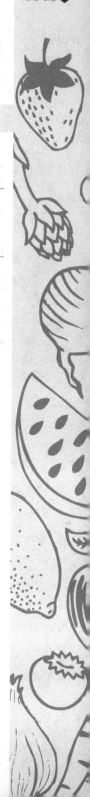

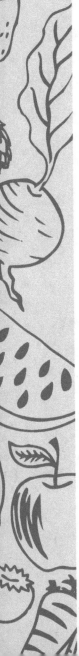

Fast, Colorful Papaya Pudding

Prep time: 8 min • **Yield:** 2 servings

Ingredients	Directions
1 large papaya, peeled and deseeded	**1** In a blender, place all the ingredients and blend until creamy. Serve.
1 large banana, peeled	
¼ teaspoon cinnamon	
2 tablespoons canned coconut milk	

Per serving: Calories 327 (From Fat 63); Fat 7g (Saturated 6g); Cholesterol 0mg; Sodium 17mg; Carbohydrate 70g (Dietary Fiber 11g); Protein 4g.

Tip: If you want the pudding cooler, pop it in the freezer for 20 minutes before serving.

Vary It! To create a thicker pudding, add 1 tablespoon of psyllium powder to the recipe. Bonus: Psyllium powder is 75 percent soluble fiber.

Tip: Decorate the top of your pudding with bananas, papaya, and coconut flakes.

Chocolate Banana Cream Pudding

Prep time: 5 min • **Yield:** 2 servings

Ingredients	Directions
4 small frozen bananas, cut into rounds	**1** In a food processor or high-speed blender, pulse the bananas, coconut milk, and cacao powder until smooth and creamy.
4 ounces full-fat coconut milk	
2 tablespoons cacao powder	**2** Serve with sliced strawberries or blueberries. Eat immediately to avoid browning.
Strawberries or blueberries, for serving	

Per serving: Calories 192 (From Fat 128); Fat 14g (Saturated 12g); Cholesterol 0mg; Sodium 10mg; Carbohydrate 16g (Dietary Fiber 2g); Protein 3g.

Tip: Cacao powder is all the rage on the raw culinary scene, so it's getting easier to obtain at health food stores or online at stores like Vitacost (www.vitacost.com).

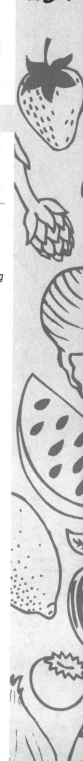

Chocolate Mousse

Prep time: 5 min • **Chilling time:** 30 min • **Yield:** 4 servings

Ingredients	Directions
1½ ripe avocados, peeled	**1** In a food processor or blender, combine all the ingredients and process or blend until smooth.
¼ cup date syrup or agave syrup	
½ cup cacao powder	**2** Chill for 30 minutes and then serve.
1 tablespoon organic vanilla	
¼ cup carob powder (optional)	

Per serving: Calories 233 (From Fat 112); Fat 12g (Saturated 4g); Cholesterol 0mg; Sodium 4mg; Carbohydrate 27g (Dietary Fiber 5g); Protein 5g.

Tip: Top with sliced strawberries for a contrasting color and taste.

Baked Treats

Most people like baking. The people who don't like baking often don't like it because baking typically requires much more precise measuring than standard cooking requires. In a stir-fry, who really cares if you have half a cup of red bell peppers instead of a quarter cup?

In baking, however, many recipes can be utterly ruined by inaccurate measuring. The recipes in this section are easy, though, because they don't contain very many ingredients and can handle substitutions and some sloppy measurements. Be the most careful with the Coconut Bread, but even there, you'll live (and your Coconut Bread will still be yummy) if your measurements aren't exactly perfect.

Each recipe in this chapter includes fruit, which ups the fiber content and overall healthiness. And, of course, fruit is low in fat. One of the healthiest desserts you can eat? Fruit! Now, if you have acid reflux, citrus is most likely out of the picture for you. Can you have a little? Maybe. Different people tolerate foods differently, but anyone who suffers from acid reflux should refrain from eating an entire orange before bedtime. Having a whole apple, though? Sure! Eating a handful of grapes next time you have a sweet tooth? Go for it! But let's face it, only a small percentage of Americans are fulfilled by fruit on a regular basis when they're trying to satisfy a sweet tooth.

When fruit alone won't cut it, reach for this book and make one of the desserts in this section. Pairing fruit with some fat and baking it was never a bad idea, even for people with acid reflux.

Blueberry Cherry Crisp

Prep time: 15 min • **Cook time:** 33–38 min • **Yield:** 8 servings

Ingredients	Directions
1 cup old-fashioned oatmeal	**1** Preheat the oven to 375 degrees. Grease a 9-x-9-inch glass dish with unsalted butter and set aside.
⅓ cup whole-wheat flour	
½ cup chopped macadamia nuts	**2** In a large bowl, combine the oatmeal, flour, and macadamia nuts. Set aside.
2 tablespoons coconut oil	
3 tablespoons butter	**3** In a small saucepan, combine the coconut oil, butter, honey, cinnamon, nutmeg, and sea salt. Heat the mixture over low heat until the butter melts, about 3 minutes. Stir the oil and butter mixture and pour it over the oatmeal mixture. Stir until the mixture becomes crumbly.
2 tablespoons honey	
1 teaspoon cinnamon	
¼ teaspoon nutmeg	
⅛ teaspoon sea salt	
4 cups frozen cherries, thawed	**4** Place the cherries and blueberries into the prepared glass dish.
2 cups frozen blueberries	**5** Spoon the oatmeal mixture over the berries. Bake for 30 to 35 minutes, or until the crisp is bubbly and the topping has browned. Serve 1½ cups per serving.

Per serving: Calories 252 (From Fat 138); Fat 16g (Saturated 7g); Cholesterol 11mg; Sodium 38mg; Carbohydrate 29g (Dietary Fiber 5g); Protein 4g.

Tip: Drizzle each serving with a bit of honey. This crisp is just as good cold the next day, so pack some in your lunchbox for a special treat.

Old-Fashioned Baked Apples with Tahini Raisin Filling

Prep time: 15 min • **Bake time:** 15 min • **Yield:** 4 servings

Ingredients	Directions
4 ripe apples	*1* Preheat the oven to 375 degrees. Lightly oil a 9-x-13-inch baking dish.
¾ cup tahini	
1 cup apple juice	*2* With a paring knife or apple corer, remove the apple core to ½ inch of the bottom of each apple. Make the holes about ¾ inch to 1 inch wide. Use a spoon to dig out the seeds. Set the apples in a shallow baking dish, top side up.
3 tablespoons raisins	
⅓ cup chopped pecans	
¼ teaspoon cinnamon	
Dash of nutmeg	*3* In a small bowl, vigorously mix the tahini and ½ cup of the apple juice. Add the raisins, pecans, cinnamon, nutmeg, and vanilla and mix the ingredients together.
Dash of vanilla	
¾ cup boiling water	
	4 Fill each cored apple with this filling.
	5 Add the boiling water to the baking pan.
	6 Pour a bit of the remaining apple juice over each apple before baking.
	7 Bake the apples for 30 to 40 minutes until tender but not mushy.
	8 Remove the apples from the oven and baste the apples several times with the remaining juices. Serve warm.

Per serving: Calories 386 (From Fat 220); Fat 24g (Saturated 3g); Cholesterol 0mg; Sodium 19mg; Carbohydrate 41g (Dietary Fiber 7g); Protein 8g.

Tip: As a traditional dessert, this recipe is especially nice to serve with a scoop of vanilla ice cream.

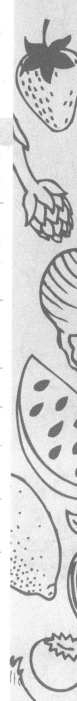

Coconut Bread

Prep time: 10 min • **Cook time:** 35–40 min • **Yield:** 10 servings

Ingredients	Directions
5 eggs	**1** Preheat the oven to 350 degrees.
1 teaspoon vanilla extract	**2** Separate 2 of the eggs.
2 teaspoons cinnamon, plus a little sprinkle to top	**3** In a medium mixing bowl, beat the 2 egg whites together with an electric mixer on high speed, until light and airy and the whites form stiff peaks, 2 to 4 minutes. Set aside.
½ teaspoon salt	
1 tablespoon baking powder	
¼ cup plus 1 teaspoon honey	**4** In a large bowl, beat together the remaining 3 whole eggs and the 2 egg yolks with an electric mixer on high speed until light and frothy, 3 to 5 minutes.
1²⁄₃ cups coconut flour	
	5 Add the vanilla, 2 teaspoons of the cinnamon, salt, baking powder, and ¼ cup of the honey; mix together on medium-high for about 1 minute.
	6 Fold the flour into the frothy egg mixture. (To fold the flour in properly, sprinkle it lightly over the top of the frothy eggs and then, using a rubber spatula, bring up the egg mixture to be gently mixed into the flour with a down-across-up-and-over motion).
	7 Fold the beaten egg whites into the mixture the same way you added the flour.
	8 Place the batter into a greased 9-x-5-inch loaf pan or an ungreased silicone bread pan.
	9 Top the dough with a sprinkle of the cinnamon and drizzle the remaining 1 teaspoon of honey on top. Bake for 35 to 40 minutes.

Per serving: Calories 150 (From Fat 46); Fat 5g (Saturated 4g); Cholesterol 93mg; Sodium 312mg; Carbohydrate 20g (Dietary Fiber 7g); Protein 6g.

Tip: Slice the bread warm or cold and spread with whipped butter and honey.

No-Bake Desserts

Is a dessert still a baked good if it isn't baked? Technically, no. But it would still be welcome at a bake sale. Go figure. The desserts in this section are about as easy as you get, with the exception of opening a candy bar wrapper. These recipes are so easy that they're great to make with kids.

For the most part, they involve loosely measuring ingredients and then rolling them together. Each recipe is high in fiber, which is great for overall health (especially if you're prone to constipation), and each is sweet without being cloying. No frosting here.

Most of the recipes in this cookbook handle substitutions well, and the same is true of this section, unless you have a nut allergy. All three of these recipes have nuts, and substituting them would be difficult. So, people with nut allergies are out of luck with this section, but people with gluten sensitivity are in good shape with the following recipes — none of these recipes contains flour.

All the ingredients are easy to find, except perhaps the turbinado sugar in the No-Bake Oat Balls. Turbinado is a golden-colored raw cane sugar with a rich aroma, somewhat like molasses. It's less processed than white granulated sugar, and the grains are much larger. They look like light-brown sparkling crystals. You can find turbinado sugar at any health food store, and some standard grocery stores.

Some nutritionists believe that turbinado is healthier than regular sugar because it's more natural, but that's up for debate. The reason it's in this book is because of the undeniable fact that it has a rich flavor that complements the oats well. If you can't find turbinado, brown sugar will do. Either way, have fun baking, er, not baking.

Almond Date Delights

Prep time: 5 min • **Cook time:** 20 min • **Yield:** 5 servings

Ingredients	Directions
2 cups almonds	*1* Preheat the oven to 375 degrees. Place the almonds on a baking sheet and roast them for about 5 minutes until brown.
1½ cups shredded coconut	
1 cup chopped pitted dates	*2* After the almonds are cooled, chop them in a food processor on pulse until the pieces are very small but not to the point of making almond butter. Remove from the processor and set aside. Wipe out the food processor bowl.
1½ cups raisins	
¼ cup water	
	3 Preheat the oven to 325 degrees. Place the coconut on a baking sheet and toast for about 10 minutes until golden brown.
	4 Remove the coconut from the oven and set aside to cool.
	5 In a food processor, blend ½ cup of the dates and ¾ cup of the raisins until the ingredients start to combine. Add a small amount of water if necessary.
	6 Gradually add the remaining dates and raisins and continue to blend into a paste. Add a little water if necessary.
	7 Add the almonds and continue to blend until the mixture forms a ball.
	8 Roll out the date mixture into about 20 balls, roughly 1 inch in diameter, and cover them with the coconut.

Per serving: Calories 765 (From Fat 365); Fat 41g (Saturated 6g); Cholesterol 0mg; Sodium 31mg; Carbohydrate 98g (Dietary Fiber 14g); Protein 19g.

No-Bake Oat Balls

Prep time: 15 min • **Yield:** 10 servings

Ingredients	Directions
1 cup turbinado sugar	**1** In a medium saucepan, combine the sugar, cocoa, milk, butter, and salt, and boil for 1 minute.
½ cup cocoa powder	
½ cup organic lowfat milk	**2** Stir the peanut butter and vanilla into the sugar mix, and remove the pan from the heat.
½ cup organic butter	
¼ teaspoon salt	**3** Place the oats in a large bowl and pour the sugar mix over the oats. Stir.
½ cup crunchy peanut butter	
1 teaspoon vanilla extract	**4** Using a spoon, drop the batter onto wax paper.
3 cups quick oats	
	5 Cool in the refrigerator for two hours.

Per serving: Calories 362 (From Fat 165); Fat 19g (Saturated 7g); Cholesterol 25mg; Sodium 66mg; Carbohydrate 45g (Dietary Fiber 5g); Protein 8g.

Making your own peanut butter

Natural peanut butter is at pretty much every grocery store these days, so that's a great option for this recipe if you don't want to make your own peanut butter. Whether you make your own peanut butter or not, opt for natural peanut butter. Natural peanut butter is lower in sugar than "unnatural" peanut butter, and doesn't have all the hydrogenated oil. If you want to make your own, follow these steps:

1. In a food processor, combine about 15 ounces roasted peanuts with 1 teaspoon salt. Optional additions are 1 to 2 teaspoons honey or 1 to 2 tablespoons peanut oil or vegetable oil.

2. Blend for 1 minute (or more if you like it smooth).

The peanut butter will last up to two months in an air-tight container in the refrigerator.

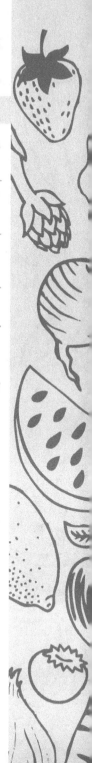

Apricot Pistachio Balls

Prep time: 30 min, plus standing • **Yield:** 36 servings

Ingredients	Directions
1 cup chopped dates	*1* Line an airtight container with parchment paper.
½ cup chopped apricots	
1 cup raw pistachios	*2* Place the dates and apricots in a food processor, and process until the fruit becomes a paste. Transfer the fruit to a medium bowl.
½ teaspoon vanilla extract	
¼ teaspoon cinnamon	*3* Add the pistachios to the food processor and process until they're finely chopped; don't process them to a paste.
	4 Add the nuts to the bowl with the fruit.
	5 Add the vanilla and cinnamon to the nut and fruit mixture. Knead the mixture together, adding a bit of water if the mixture seems dry.
	6 Wet your hands with water. Form the fruit and nut mixture into ¾-inch balls and place them in the container lined with parchment paper. Let the balls stand until they're set, about 1 hour.

Per serving: Calories 68 (From Fat 31); Fat 4g (Saturated 1g); Cholesterol 0mg; Sodium 2mg; Carbohydrate 10g (Dietary Fiber 1g); Protein 1g.

Tip: Store leftovers in an airtight container at room temperature for 3 to 4 days.

Part IV
Solutions for Specific Situations

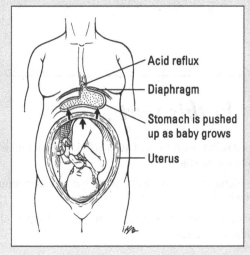

Illustration by Kathryn Born

Get a guide to eating out in a free article at www.dummies.com/extras/acidrefluxdiet.

In this part . . .

✔ Find acid reflux–friendly food at almost any restaurant and pack for any outing.

✔ From pregnancy to your golden years, manage acid reflux no matter where you are in life.

✔ Find out about surgical options when diet and lifestyle changes and medications don't work.

Chapter 15

Finding Safe Dishes When You're Eating Out

Controlling food at home is pretty easy, but controlling it outside the home can be tough. Eating reflux friendly when you step outside your home is possible, though, and with a little planning and knowledge, it's a piece of cake. However, it likely doesn't include any cake at all, so don't get your hopes up.

Packing Heat: Bringing Foods When You're Away from Home

A few minutes of planning is worth a roll of antacids. When you know you're going to be away from home for a while, you can pack a meal or snack so that you don't have to worry about finding something safe to eat.

If you make enough food for meals at home, you'll have leftovers for lunch at work or school. Just make sure you have the proper containers — brown bags, cloth bags, Tupperware, a thermos.

Pretty much anything that's not on the list of reflux trigger foods (see Chapter 4 for a list of foods that aggravate acid reflux) can make a decent snack. Just be sure it's not very high in fat and, if it is, keep the portion small. Here are some great snacks that can keep your reflux at bay:

✔ Avocados

✔ Bananas

- Hummus
- Leafy greens
- Lowfat dairy
- Melon
- Nuts (just watch your portions — limit yourself to a handful or two)
- Oatmeal
- Rice
- Rice cakes
- Tofu
- Veggies (cooked or raw)

An ounce of prevention is worth a pound of cure

Your goal is to prevent reflux from occurring, and a key part of prevention is planning. How many times have you been stressed out at work, hungry as heck, and you have nothing to eat? By the time you get out of that four-hour meeting that was supposed to be two hours you're famished, and maybe you eat three times as much of whatever's in front of you, or roll through a fast food lane and supersize your curly fries? This isn't good for maintaining a healthy weight, and healthy weight is important for keeping acid reflux away.

Plus, if your blood sugar is low, which happens when the human body goes too long without eating, you're more likely to eat anything that's in front of you. That could mean all kinds of acid reflux villains, like spaghetti loaded with acidic tomato sauce, or nachos covered in tomatoes, raw onions, greasy cheese, fatty beef, scorching jalapeños, and garlicky salsa.

If you plan your meals and snacks for work, school, and trips and if you think ahead about restaurant choices, you'll be less likely to make hunger-driven decisions. You'll feel in control, and feeling in control will reduce stress. And what happens when your stress levels are lower? You're less likely to have heartburn.

Remember: To make meal packing easier, keep the refrigerator clean. Get rid of that clutter — the pickle jar with one lone pickle in it or the container of take-out food from last week. You'll have an easier time seeing what you have, which will make planning smoother. Do the same for cabinets and cupboards.

Check out Chapter 6 for tips on how to plan meals for the week. Because you'll already have all that food made that you know is good for your acid reflux, you'll have ample choices on hand for lunches, picnics, trips, and more.

Finding Reflux-Friendly Foods on the Menu

This book is full of easy, tasty recipes that will help tame your heartburn, but even an easy recipe still involves doing dishes. Blah! For those days when you don't want to cook or clean, or when you're away from home, you can take your reflux-friendly diet to restaurants. Some restaurants will have more choices for you than others, but you should be able to find something you'll enjoy almost anywhere.

In this section, we break it down by type of cuisine, so you know what to look for on the menu.

Chinese

When it comes to Chinese food, the big challenge if you have acid reflux is that a lot of Chinese meals are fried, include meat, and are greasy and spicy. That's not a big problem, though, because most chefs at Chinese restaurants can easily adapt your order.

Most Chinese dishes are made one at a time and can be customized. Exceptions include soups and sauces, which are usually premade. Avoid or have very small amounts of greasy and/or spicy soups and sauces. Otherwise, ask your server for adjustments to your meal.

Most vegetarian meals will be fine for your acid reflux. Just ask the server to make it mild instead of medium or high spice. If the meal shows up very greasy, eat a small quantity of it. *Remember:* Excess grease promotes acid reflux.

A lot of Chinese food has garlic and onion. Garlic and onion are much worse for acid reflux if they're raw, and that's rare in Chinese food. Still, the garlic and onion in Chinese food is often very lightly cooked and could activate your heartburn. Avoid dishes that make garlic and onion the star of the dish. For instance, garlic eggplant probably isn't a good choice.

Mexican

Mexican food isn't quite as easy as Chinese food, but you still have lots of options. The main problem will be salsa, because it's tomato based and many styles of salsa also include raw onion, garlic, and spice. So, you may have to skip the salsa all together or have a small amount.

The avocados in guacamole are good for digestion even though they're high fat. However, guacamole often includes raw onion and garlic. Ask your server for guacamole without onion and garlic — most of the time, the staff will be able to accommodate you. Mexican food often includes rogue raw onions and jalapeños, so ask your server to leave them off anything you order.

Beer and margaritas are tasty with Mexican food, but try to avoid them because alcohol is an acid-reflux no-no.

Follow all these tips, go easy on the meat, keep your portions small or moderate, and you'll be fine at any Mexican restaurant.

Italian

Yes, the tomato sauce rampant at most Italian restaurants is a problem for the acid reflux prone, and so is the ample use of garlic. Also challenging: the fact that wine tastes so lovely with Italian food, yet triggers acid reflux. Avoid the alcohol, or drink less than usual.

To avoid tomato sauces, try pesto or Alfredo sauces (small portions, though — all the fat in Alfredo sauce can trigger reflux, and pesto tends to be heavy on garlic).

Even if you steer clear of acid reflux foods, just eating too much can lead to a yucky night. Wherever and whatever you eat, keep your portions small or moderate.

Japanese

Folks, we have a winner! Japanese food is great for people wanting to avoid acid reflux. Just stay away from the deep-fried items, such as tempura. Avoiding fried items is easy because there are lots of fresh, non-fried offerings at Japanese restaurants.

Avoid the alcohol, as usual (sorry, no Saki bombers — or at least not as many as usual), and avoid the wasabi. This extremely hot paste is great for cleaning out the sinuses, but it may also activate your reflux.

Thai

Thai food is similar to Chinese, but it's slightly easier because Thai food is usually less greasy than Chinese food. As with Chinese food, ask for it mild instead of medium or hot.

Diners

At diners, avoid meals that have big quantities of meat (a big ol' burger isn't a good choice). Also avoid fried foods — that side of french fries won't help you.

Most diners have salads (just skip the raw onion), soups, sandwiches, and plenty of other foods that will fare well with your sensitive tract. If you order dessert (so tempting when diners have their own baked goods), remember to have a fairly small portion so you don't take in too much fat.

Fast food

At fast-food restaurants, skip or eat less of any meal that makes meat the prime star. Skip or eat less of the fries and anything else that's fried. Keep dessert portions small. Be mindful of how much fat you're having overall, because excess fat increases reflux. Almost all fast-food places have salads and grilled chicken sandwiches these days, so those could be good choices.

Even if you don't have something super "healthy," you'll be okay as long as you keep your quantity small and don't have that type of food too often. If you're having fast food more than a few times a month, it's probably too often, unless what you're ordering is healthy.

Chapter 16

From Pregnancy to the Golden Years: Managing Acid Reflux in Special Communities

. . . .

In This Chapter

▶ Handling acid reflux when you're pregnant

▶ Helping your child cope with acid reflux

▶ Managing acid reflux as you age

. . . .

A cid reflux is stronger for some people than for others, and more frequent for some people than for others, but for the most part, acid reflux is acid reflux. It burns, it's uncomfortable, it can be painful, and it can be dangerous. That much is consistent across all demographics. Some groups of people, however, experience acid reflux a little differently and have special considerations. Pregnant women, babies, children, and seniors have some things to think about that are unique to their population. In this chapter, we address these considerations, in case you fall into one of these groups, now or in the future.

When You're Pregnant

As if women don't have enough to deal with when they're pregnant (for example, breast discomfort, tiny kicking feet, and out-of-whack hormones), a majority of them end up having acid reflux as well. Who doesn't want to be woken up by liquid fire pushing up her throat when she's already uncomfortable because of the human being she's carrying around? Sorry, bearers of humanity — at least half of you experience acid reflux. The acid reflux appears at different points of pregnancy for different women, and some have it the whole way through. It usually gets worse as the pregnancy develops, especially after 27 weeks. In general, if you had acid reflux often *before* pregnancy, it will get worse *during* pregnancy. Some women who have never had acid reflux or who rarely have it are surprised to develop it.

Why is this condition so common during pregnancy? Pregnancy hormones slow the digestive system. No one knows why. But regardless, those pesky hormones tell the muscles of the esophagus to move more slowly than usual, and this can make it easier for acid to go north. The hormone change can also relax the lower esophageal sphincter (LES).

Another reason for increased acid reflux: As the baby gets bigger, it pushes against the stomach in a game of "there's not room for the both of us." That pressure forces acid from the stomach up the esophagus, and casualties ensue. Hello, acid reflux. Figure 16-1 shows the relationship between the growing uterus and the esophagus.

Figure 16-1:
As the uterus expands throughout pregnancy, it pushes on the stomach and can force acid up the esophagus.

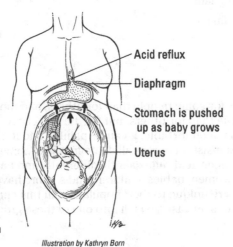

Illustration by Kathryn Born

Treatment options for pregnant women with acid reflux are similar to treatment options for anyone else. Focus on

- ✔ **Diet:** See all of Part III for recipes.

- ✔ **Lifestyle changes:** In particular, you want to focus on eating smaller, more frequent meals, and not eating near bedtime. (See Chapter 7 for more on lifestyle changes.)

✔ **Antacids:** Pregnant women can use nonprescription antacids, such as Rolaids or Tums, but ask your doctor first.

Pregnant women should *not* take antacids that contain sodium bicarbonate, which can cause fluid retention. Pregnant women *can* take antacids that contain calcium carbonate. Talk to your doctor before you start taking any antacid, regardless of ingredients.

If diet and lifestyle changes and nonprescription antacids don't decrease the acid reflux, talk to your doctor about the prescription drug sucralfate. Your doctor may recommend acid reducers or proton pump inhibitors (PPIs), which reduce stomach acid levels.

The silver lining for pregnancy and acid reflux? Heartburn usually decreases or goes away completely when the baby is born. Thanks, little guy.

When You're Pint Size

Babies spit up. It happens. Kids throw up, too. But when that spit-up and upchuck occurs too harshly or too often, it could be a sign of acid reflux. How do you know? By looking for certain symptoms. Symptoms of acid reflux in babies and kids include the following:

✔ Frequent vomiting not associated with stomach bug or nausea

✔ Persistent cough not associated with cold, flu, or allergy

✔ Having a hard time eating, such as crying, choking, gagging, or looking like it's painful to swallow

In the following sections, we cover acid reflux in babies and kids, offering tips that can help ease the symptoms and get to the root cause.

Acid reflux in babies

Most of the time, infants with acid reflux are otherwise healthy, and the acid reflux isn't related to other conditions. However, some infants have problems with their muscles, nerves, and/or brains, or have underdeveloped digestive systems. Even in these cases, a majority of infants outgrow their acid reflux before their first birthday.

In the meantime, the following tips may help your poor baby:

✔ Thicken bottle milk with cereal (but ask your doctor first).

✔ Try to feed her solid food (again, ask your doctor first).

✔ Alter your baby's feeding schedule.

✔ Keep her upright at least 30 minutes after a feeding. (We know — you want her to go to sleep. Sorry. At least keep her head elevated in your arms; she doesn't have to be sitting straight up to dissuade acid reflux. Even slight elevation helps).

✔ Avoid moving her around much after feeding. (No jumpers! No spazzy older cousins getting their wish to finally hold the baby.)

Reducing stomach acid helps some adult sufferers of acid reflux, but researchers aren't sure whether decreasing stomach acid lessens reflux in infants.

Acid reflux in kids

The causes of acid reflux in kids include foods, beverages, medications, eating too much, being overweight, or being constipated. All this can increase pressure on the LES and lead to acid reflux. If you think your child has acid reflux, take him to the doctor. Usually a doctor can make a diagnosis just from your account and/or your child's, but every now and then, the doctor may recommend tests. Your child won't like these tests, so you may want to advertise how awesome it is that he gets to miss school. Plus, he'll have a pretty wild story for his friends the next day.

Tests for kids who may have acid reflux or other conditions include the following:

✔ **Upper GI endoscopy:** An endoscopy uses an *endoscope,* which is a long, thin, instrument with a light and camera at one end. This thin tube goes down the child's mouth and into his esophagus. The child's throat is numbed first. The doctor (a gastroenterologist) uses the endoscope camera to look at the esophagus, the stomach, and the top part of the small intestine.

✔ **pH probe:** This procedure is a little like an upper GI endoscopy, but it uses a much smaller instrument, and the procedure lasts longer. The child swallows a long, thin tube and has to keep this tube in the esophagus for 24 hours. The process doesn't hurt, but of course no kid will like it. The tip of the probe hovers near the lower esophagus and measures stomach acid. This procedure can also help diagnose whether the digestive problem your child may have is causing breathing problems.

✔ **Upper GI series/barium swallow:** This is an X-ray that can identify if parts of the digestive tract are too narrow or are obstructed. The child swallows a milkshake of *barium* (it sounds scary, but it's safe). The barium highlights the esophagus, the stomach, and the top part of the small intestine and allows the radiologist to see if the barium regurgitates, if the stomach empties, or if there is a hiatal hernia or an esophageal stricture.

✔ **Gastric emptying:** You may be thinking that your child already does enough gastric emptying, if his acid reflux is causing him to throw up. Well, this is a different kind. Instead of the contents coming up, they go down. Like the upper GI series/barium swallow, this test requires the child to eat a radioactive tracer mixed with milk or food; a radiologist uses a Geiger counter like X-ray device to track its journey. This will tell the doctor if the child's stomach empties too slowly. Tummies that empty too slowly can cause acid reflux.

Here are some ways you can try to decrease acid reflux in kids:

✔ Follow the diet in this book.

✔ Elevate the head of your child's bed by propping up his mattress a little, or by propping up the headboard itself.

✔ Don't let the child lie down until at least two hours after his last meal.

✔ Consider serving several small meals and snacks throughout the day, instead of three big meals.

✔ Help your child to lose weight if he's overweight.

If these strategies don't work well enough, take your child back to the doctor and ask about antacids and prescription medications. Antacids are generally safe, even for kids, but high doses can cause diarrhea, and who wants to replace one digestive problem with another? In addition, high doses of antacids may cause difficulties with absorption of vitamins needed to help kids thrive — so check with your doctor before you keep giving your kid over-the-counter antacids.

Chronic high doses of Mylanta or Maalox can thin bones or cause vitamin deficiency. So, if your doctor suggests that you give your child these medications, follow the directions exactly and don't depend on their use long term. Changing diet and lifestyle is much better.

In some cases, surgery is needed to treat acid reflux in kids, but this is very rare. The most common surgery for kids who have acid reflux is the Nissen fundoplication (turn to Chapter 17 for more information). Very few kids will need this surgery. If your doctor recommends it, make sure you understand the risks, and be sure you've exhausted all other options.

Every surgery — even low-risk, common surgeries like fundoplication — introduce the risk of infection, bleeding, perforation, and anesthesia complications. All the more reason to put off surgery unless you and your doctor are sure it's absolutely necessary.

When You're Older and Wiser

Acid reflux is more common in senior populations than in other demographics, but statistics vary as to just how common it is.

Just as acid reflux is different in infants than it is in kids, acid reflux is different in younger adults than it is in older adults. For one thing, acid reflux in older adults can be much more dangerous and lead to more complications. The main symptom of gastroesophageal reflux disease (GERD) for younger adults is usually regurgitation. For the older and wiser among us, however, common symptoms can also include

- ✔ Asthma
- ✔ Chest pain
- ✔ Chronic cough
- ✔ Dental problems
- ✔ Indigestion or upset stomach
- ✔ Stricture with dysphagia (food getting trapped in the esophagus)
- ✔ Vomiting

Older people with GERD may have upper-gastrointestinal bleeding, esophageal strictures, Barrett's esophagus (see Chapter 3), or esophageal cancer as a result. The most common GERD complication for seniors is *esophagitis* (inflammation or shallow ulcers of the esophagus). Esophagitis is about three times more common in the elderly than in younger populations.

Because GERD is more dangerous for older people than younger people, older folks and their doctors need to treat it more aggressively. The treatment options are similar as for other groups: diet, lifestyle changes, medication, and surgery.

Chapter 17

When Diet and Alternative Therapies Don't Cut It: Surgical Options

. . . .

In This Chapter

▶ Looking at procedures that treat acid reflux

▶ Considering the acid reflux–cancer connection

▶ Preparing for surgery

▶ Recovering from surgery

. . . .

So, altering your diet and lifestyle didn't cut it. If that's the case, you're not alone. It's estimated that some 12 million Americans with gastroesophageal reflux disease (GERD) don't improve enough with lifestyle changes or medications.

Many times doctors can manage reflux with long-term use of medications, but sometimes either the meds aren't completely suppressing the reflux (doctors call this *breakthrough symptoms*) or you just don't want to take a daily medication. Or, maybe you've developed a complication of reflux, such as a stricture, Barrett's esophagus, or cancer. For a variety of reasons, you and your doctor may decide it's time to consider medical procedures such as new endoscopic anti reflux procedures, or even surgery.

In this chapter, we walk you through the procedures that treat GERD. We also cover the cancer connection, and fill you in on treatments. Finally, we give you the info you need before donning that hospital gown, and tell you what to expect from your recovery.

Everyone with acid reflux hopes they can manage their condition with lifestyle modifications and medication alone, but sometimes that's just not in the cards. Fortunately, there are options that can bring you relief.

Last Resort: Surgery

This book is loaded with advice on how to reduce acid reflux symptoms. But the fact is, you may follow every tip to the letter and still feel the pain of acid reflux. If you've done everything you can to modify your lifestyle, worked with your doctor to try a variety of medications, and you're still suffering, it may be time to consider surgery. Nobody has surgery for the fun of it — unless you're Joan Rivers, surgery is always a last resort. But the good news is, when it comes to treating GERD, there are surgical options that can bring relief. In this section, we give you a rundown of the main types of surgery you might have to treat acid reflux, as well as Barrett's esophagus and esophageal cancer.

The mainstay: Nissen fundoplication

The most common surgical procedure — and one that has been around for years — is the Nissen fundoplication, which has about an 85 percent success rate in relieving reflux symptoms and healing inflammation of the esophagus.

The procedure involves wrapping the upper stomach, or *fundus,* around the lower part of the esophagus. Think of it like a hot dog (the esophagus) in a hot dog bun (the stomach) — hold the relish and mustard. This procedure compresses the lower end of the esophagus, and this compression prevents reflux. The higher pressure in the lower esophageal sphincter (LES) area occurs only when you need it — when food is in your stomach and the food-filled wrapped stomach "smooshes" the esophagus.

There is a lot of variety in terms of how surgeons do their Nissens, including how tightly the "bun" wraps the "hot dog," whether the "hot dog" sits atop the "bun" or is completely enveloped by it, and the length of "hot dog" and "bun" involved. All the procedures have different names, but at the heart they're derivatives of the classic Nissen. The Nissen fundoplication also may be performed *open* (with a traditional surgical incision) or *closed* (via laparoscopy). Laparoscopic ("lap") Nissens have similar results to conventional open surgery, with shorter recovery times.

A Nissen fundoplication isn't perfect. After surgery, a disappointed 10 percent to 65 percent of patients still require some form of antiacid medication. However, the reflux is mostly less severe than in the pre-op state. And surgery carries, as always, the usual risk of complications, including bleeding, infection, perforation, and risks from anesthesia.

If you're thinking that 10 percent to 65 percent is a huge range, you're right, but that's the data. Some studies select for folks with good response to medications, and they're more likely to have good outcomes. The people with breakthrough symptoms despite maximum drugs tend to have disappointing outcomes. Doctors think it may have something to do with having a sensitive esophagus, not the quantity or acidity of the material getting through. Bottom line: No procedure works for everyone.

Side effects of a Nissen include the gas-bloat syndrome (see "Long-term changes," later in this chapter). In addition, a tightly wrapped Nissen may cause difficulty swallowing in an esophagus that moves well. It's important to have the *motility* (movement) test of the esophagus before having this surgery — if the esophagus itself (in addition to the LES) is weak, it's a recipe for disaster to then have a Nissan done and have your esophagus fail to get Aunt Mary's fried chicken all the way through the wrap to your stomach.

Some new endoscopic methods are being developed that tighten the sphincter with a suture or staple placed from the inside. Our advice: Don't be an early adopter on a new endoscopy or surgical procedure unless you're out of options. Sometimes new procedures have significant complications and end up being discontinued. Let somebody else be the guinea pig, if possible, and stick with the tried and true. Or wait until the new technique has some mileage under its tires.

Cooking the esophagus: The Stretta procedure

The Stretta radiofrequency system, approved by the Food and Drug Administration (FDA) in 2000, uses radiofrequency (RF) energy to increase collagen contraction at the sphincter and to decrease nerve sensitivity to acid at the lower end of the esophagus. It's sort of like cooking the lower esophagus and esophageal sphincter via microwaves.

The gastroenterologist does an upper endoscopy (technically called an esophagogastroduodenoscopy, or EGD) and measures the distance from the person's teeth to the junction of the esophagus and stomach. Then the gastroenterologist withdraws the endoscope and inserts the RF catheter. This complicated catheter is a 4-foot-long slender tube that has an inflatable balloon at the end. Four additional slender catheters run down the central catheter's sides and end alongside the balloon. The peripheral tubes have retractable short needles. The balloon is inflated to press the needle tubes against the esophageal lining, the needles are advanced out, and then the gastroenterologist "cooks" the esophagus in those areas using RF through the needles for about a minute. The needles are retracted, the balloon is deflated, and the catheter is repositioned to a different level in the esophagus. Usually, a patient gets about 60 total zaps over about 30 minutes.

The Stretta procedure has a long track record. The ten-year data, released in 2013, were good, but not perfect. Of the 99 study participants with refractory GERD followed for ten years, 41 percent no longer required the medications they were taking pre-Stretta. That means 59 percent were still on meds.

Stretta is not complication free, but it's pretty safe. Serious complications — such as esophageal perforation and aspiration pneumonia — have been reported, but complications were mainly modest in more than 1,400 patients participating in 20 studies. The most common complications were temporary upper abdominal pain in 66 percent of patients, chest pain in 15 percent, ulcers in the esophagus in 4 percent, and difficult or painful swallowing in 3 percent.

Magnetic attraction: New procedures with magnets

One of the newest procedures for treating GERD involves magnets. The LINX Reflux Management System is a bracelet of titanium-coated beads with a magnetic core. A surgeon does a laparoscopic surgery, which includes making a small incision in the upper abdomen to gain access to the area at the top of the stomach and bottom of the esophagus, the area just below the sternum. Then she places the bracelet around the lower end of the esophagus. Patients are usually sent home the same day.

The LINX device works just like a magnet — it attracts opposite sides of the esophagus together to close it up. This closure prevents gastric contents from moving up the esophagus. Yes, the magnets are powerful, but they can pull apart to allow normal swallowed material to make it into the stomach.

Early data on the device look good, but — as you can probably guess by now — it's not perfect. During early clinical studies on this new device, 100 patients who had severe GERD for an average of 13 years and experienced around 80 heartburn attacks a week were examined before the procedure and 12 months after the procedure. In just over half the patients, the amount of time that the esophagus was exposed to acid fell by at least one-half; these patients reported that their quality of life improved as well. Three-quarters of the patients experienced side effects, the most common being difficulty swallowing, which in some cases took six months or more to resolve. The second most common side effect was pain. In five patients, the device had to be removed.

Don't ask for a LINX if you have allergies to metals such as iron, nickel, titanium, or stainless steel. Also, after you have it put in, you can never again have a magnetic resonance imaging (MRI) scan because the uber-powerful magnets in an MRI scanner don't play well with the metal in the LINX. The LINX system is also problematic for patients receiving electrical implants such as defibrillators or pacemakers or undergoing insertion of metallic implants in the abdomen. The LINX device is also not recommended in patients with large hiatal hernias — *large* here is defined as bigger than 3 cm.

The LINX device is still very new, which means it hasn't been tested by time or large numbers of patients.

Never be an early adopter of new technology unless you have no other option.

Endoscopic mucosal resection

If you have Barrett's esophagus (see Chapter 3), you may need a surgical procedure known as endoscopic mucosal resection (EMR). EMR is a way for doctors to chop off a chunk of esophagus deep down to the submucosa. It allows doctors to remove and send to pathologists hunks of tissue rather than mere crumbs of tissue. These large tissue specimens can be examined by pathologists to determine the type and depth of the abnormality, and whether adequate surrounding tissue (called *margin*) was removed.

EMR is used when the endoscopist sees a *nodule,* or bump, in an area of Barrett's esophagus that may be an early esophageal cancer or an area of high-grade *dysplasia.*

Dysplasia is diagnosed when the pathologist sees angry-looking cells through his microscope. These unusual or atypical cells are considered to be the first step toward cancer. Dysplasia comes as low, moderate, or high grade, with severe dysplasia being indistinguishable from cancer.

If cancer is present, the depth of the invasion will let the doctor know if he treated it successfully or whether surgery to remove the esophagus is necessary.

EMR may be combined with radiofrequency ablation (RFA; see Chapter 3) for folks with a combination of nodules and Barrett's, but not in the same setting. That's just too much trauma on the esophagus: You don't want your doctor to chop out a hunk of esophagus and then fry the rest of the esophagus in one fell swoop. Besides being unpleasantly painful, this combination would increase the risk of a perforation to the esophagus.

In EMR, the surgeon uses a special short plastic sleeve (called an *endoscopic resection cap*) on the tip of an endoscope to suck up the offending nodule. The surgeon then deploys a rubber band around the neck of this faux polyp. He uses a snare around the "polyp" and applies current through the wire snare that acts like a sharp knife and slices off the tissue. Multiple bands can be placed and multiple chunks can be removed. Broad areas of the esophagus lining can be stripped off in this process.

EMR takes a lot of training, and most gastroenterologists haven't had it. If EMR is needed, many patients are sent to *teaching hospitals* (medical centers affiliated with medical training programs) to have this specialized technique done. If your local gastroenterologist plans to do EMR, or any advanced technique, it's fair game to ask him about his experience and training for the new technique. If he blows off your concerns, it's second-opinion time. Not all gastroenterologists do all advanced procedures well — you just can't be an expert in everything.

Esophagectomy

Because of the anatomy of the esophagus, passing through the *mediastinum* (the area in your mid chest that includes the heart and the trachea and main bronchi to both lungs), taking out just a segment of the esophagus when you have esophageal cancer isn't an option. And the esophagus, not enveloped in a capsule of connective tissue as so many other organs are, passes cancer to lymph nodes and to the other important structures in the mediastinum very early on.

Meet the *esophagectomy,* removal of the esophagus. Yes, it's drastic, but it's done with the intent to cure, and if it's offered to you, it's because the surgeons and oncologists believe that it'll work.

Before offering an esophagectomy, your gastroenterologist, oncologist, or surgeon will do what is called *staging* of the cancer, to determine whether it has spread to lymph nodes or other organs. This may include a CT scan of the chest and an endoscopic ultrasound. An endoscopic ultrasound is where you have an upper endoscopy (of the esophagus area) with a special endoscope. The endoscope has a tip that takes ultrasound pictures, and that can take deep-needle biopsies through the esophagus wall and out into lymph nodes and surrounding structures through the scope.

You may not be offered the surgery if you have other medical conditions such as poor functioning of the heart and lungs. But even if your lymph nodes are involved, sometimes the oncologists will give you chemotherapy or radiation to see if the lymph nodes can be shrunk to normal size, thereby making you a surgical candidate.

For an esophagectomy, the surgeons remove the entire esophagus, from where it starts at the base of the neck to where it attaches to the top of the stomach. They then mobilize your stomach, freeing it from the connective tissue that has held it in place your entire life, and advance it up through your mediastinum and attach it to the pharynx (the back of the throat). When you swallow, instead of food entering the esophagus for a trip down to the stomach, it's there immediately. Your stomach is up in your chest. And, we hope, your cancer is cured.

Somewhat surprisingly, you can have a relatively normal life after the surgery. Most patients who have had esophagectomy are happy to be alive, although most continue to have issues with food regurgitation, shortness of breath, and some diarrhea.

What to Expect from Surgery or Advanced Endoscopy Techniques

When it comes time for your surgery, you'll be instructed to eat nothing after midnight the night before and to stop drinking water or fluids four hours before the surgery. Your anesthesiologist wants to make sure that your stomach is empty and you won't regurgitate anything up into your lungs while you're asleep on the table.

On your arrival to the hospital, after you fill out all that pesky paperwork, a nurse will take you back to a pre-op room where, in no particular order, you'll sign a consent form, be given one of those snazzy backless gowns to change into, and have an IV started in your arm. The IV (short for intravenous) is a catheter into a vein in your arm attached to a bag of fluid, allowing your anesthesiologist to give you the happy drugs for your procedure. You'll also meet your anesthesiologist, who will check your teeth and ability to open your mouth, and ask you about any prior experiences and side effects of anesthesia.

Then it's show time! You'll be wheeled back to the operating room (OR) or to the endoscopy suite, where your doctors and nurses await your arrival with bated breath. Regardless of which location you're sent to, before you head off to sleep, your doctor will lead a *timeout*, stating out loud who you are, what you're there for, and any specific medical problems or anticipated issues he may have. The rules are that anyone may object at this point, and things will come to a screeching halt. If you're not there for a vasectomy, now's the time to object.

Then you're asleep, and the doctor's magic begins.

All surgeries differ from patient to patient, hospital to hospital, and surgeon to surgeon, so we can't tell you for sure what your particular surgical experience will be like. If you have questions about what to expect from surgery, be sure to talk with your doctor beforehand. She should be able to answer all your questions and allay any concerns you may have.

All About Recovery

Recovery from surgery depends on the type of surgery you've had. In this section, we let you know what to expect.

What you can eat after surgery

What you can eat after surgery depends on the procedure you had:

- **Nissen fundoplication or LINX:** If you had a Nissen fundoplication or LINX, you may eat a normal, albeit anti-reflux diet. You may need to chew solids thoroughly, taking sips of fluid after each bite, to ensure that the food makes it through the area of high pressure in the lower esophagus that has been surgically created. Your physician has likely made the procedure good and tight, to make you one of the folks who need no supplemental reflux medications. So, for a while, expect that chunks of bread and lumps of meat may cause some feelings of hesitancy in your esophagus.

- **Stretta procedure or EMR:** Depending on the amount of tissue removed or the amount of burn during the procedure, this sucker can smart. The esophagus has great nerves, and after the anesthesia wears off, this may feel like the mother of all reflux episodes.

  You'll be instructed to take the highest dose of a proton-pump inhibitor (PPI) twice daily for one to three months, to help the abused tissue to heal without scar. Your doctor may prescribe a mix of Lidocaine (a swallowable Novocain) and antacid, and you'll be on a liquid diet (no acidic juices — ouch!) for a day, followed by a soft and bland diet for a week. Finally, you need to watch out for bleeding (bloody vomit or black stools), or a sudden increase in chest pain (which may signal a perforation), or a fever (which may indicate an *abscess,* or infection).

- **Esophagectomy:** If you have an esophagectomy, the surgeon will surgically insert a flexible straw-diameter feeding tube directly into your *jejunum* (a part of the small intestine) through the abdominal wall to support nutrition as you recover. This will usually be done during the esophagectomy surgery. The surgeon needs to make sure that where she sewed the pharynx to the stomach (up in the neck) doesn't leak before she can allow you to eat normally. You'll get liquid feedings through this tube for several days until your bowels recover from the insult and start moving normally.

Any time a bowel operation causes surgeons to handle or cut the gastro-intestinal tract, the bowels become temporarily paralyzed, a condition called *ileus.*

The tube feedings will start around two days after the surgery, as a trickle of feedings through the tube, increasing slowly each day for three to five days. The slow advance is to allow the ileus to resolve — your doctors don't want you to feel nauseated, vomit, and disrupt your stitches.

A few days after surgery (it's up to your surgeon), you'll be asked to swallow a barium solution. Barium is a thick milkshake of X-ray contrast. When X-rays of your neck are taken, any of the barium solution that leaks out can be seen on the X-ray. The goal is to prove that there is no leakage into the tissues of your neck.

When your doctor has determined that there is no leakage, you'll be on a liquid diet by mouth for about two more weeks. Then you'll move on to solid foods. Your doctor will have you eat foods that are easy to digest (low fat, low fiber).

How long it takes to heal

Healing from a Nissen fundoplication or LINX can be fast, especially if it was done laparoscopically. Some patients may be sent home the day after surgery, once they have proven that they can swallow food without issues.

Healing from a Stretta or EMR can be slow; it really depends on how much tissue needed to be burned or removed. And because the esophagus tends to have a lot of nerves, it can be painful. Be aggressive in managing the acid with medications, and be gentle with foods by eating things that are soft or nonacidic. Most folks feel fine within a week.

Healing from an esophagectomy is slow — measured in years. Most patients heal one to two years after surgery, but even after three or more years, a substantial number of long-term survivors still experience issues such as difficult or painful swallowing, shortness of breath, and reflux. Eighty-six percent of esophagectomy patients are stable or improved at five years.

Long-term changes

If you've had a Nissen fundoplication, or any other surgery or endoscopic procedure to tighten the lower end of the esophagus, be aware of *gas-bloat syndrome*. Gas-bloat syndrome is a sensation of gas and fullness, yet being unable to belch. When your doctor tightens the lower end of the esophagus, the intent is to keep solids and liquid down in the stomach where they belong. Unfortunately, that means air will fail to escape as well. Gas bloat is seen more often when the wrap is tight, which is in fact what you want. Gas bloat can be a side effect of a well-done procedure.

If you get gas-bloat syndrome, you should avoid carbonated beverages or drinking through straws. Simethecone or charcoal tablets may relieve some of the gas, but studies supporting this aren't available. Evaluation of stomach emptying, via a nuclear-medicine gastric-emptying test or a *smart pill* (a tiny camera) may lead to the use of medications that help gas bloat syndrome, but those medications have side effects, such as irritability, anxiety, and depression.

Certainly esophagectomy causes long-term changes in health and lifestyle, however, being alive trumps the alternative. Long-term issues include *anastomotic stricture* (narrowing of the junction of the stomach and the pharynx in the neck). This occurs in up to 40 percent of patients and requires dilation (sometimes repeatedly every couple months) by the gastroenterologist during an endoscopy. Symptoms of the anastomotic stricture are painful or difficult swallowing.

Other issues after esophagectomy include *dumping syndrome* (too rapid stomach emptying with sweats, nausea, and diarrhea), *postprandial hypoglycemia* (low blood sugar after eating), and slow gastric emptying with regurgitation of stomach contents into the mouth. Dumping occurs in up to 50 percent of patients following esophagectomy. Twenty-five percent of patients experience postprandial hypoglycemia, and an additional 50 percent have delayed gastric emptying. Some people have several of these issues and may experience both rapid and delayed emptying at times.

The management of these post-operative issues with the function of the stomach in the chest require great attention to diet: Avoid simple sugars, and eat frequent small meals. However, although management is tough, being alive still wins.

Part V
The Part of Tens

In this part . . .

- ✔ Change your eating habits.
- ✔ Modify your kitchen.
- ✔ Separate the myths about acid reflux from the facts.
- ✔ Recognize the benefits of life without acid reflux.

Chapter 18

Ten (Or So) Simple Ways to Change Your Eating Habits

In This Chapter

▶ Realizing what you want to change

▶ Setting goals

▶ Giving yourself options

▶ Adjusting to change

*T*he advice in this chapter can work for any diet, whether you're vegetarian, gluten free, or just reducing calories. The very first step is to decide that you want to change your habits. After you make that decision, the sky's the limit! Have you decided? Of course you have — you bought this book!

Writing Down Your Goals

You aren't changing your diet for nothing. What are the goals you'd like to meet? Here are some of the many possibilities:

✔ You want to reduce your acid reflux (both the frequency and the severity).

✔ You want to reduce your heartburn.

✔ You want to reduce your chances of getting Barrett's esophagus, or of making it worse if you already have it.

✔ You want to reduce your risk of illnesses associated with acid reflux, such as asthma or esophageal cancer.

✔ You want to feel better overall.

✔ You want to lose weight.

✔ You want to sleep better.

✔ You want to learn more about what bothers your reflux and what doesn't.

Write your own list of goals. Below that, write what you would like to feel. For instance, "I want to feel healthy overall, and to either never have reflux again, or have it only a few times a year. I want to feel good and not have to worry about reflux."

Hold onto that piece of paper for at least the first few months of your eating regime. You may want to put it somewhere you'll see it all the time, such as on the refrigerator, your desk, or your dashboard. If you want it somewhere more private, keep it in a file on your computer or put it in your sock drawer. Wherever you keep your list of goals, look at it occasionally to remind yourself why you're making the changes you're making.

Sharing Your Goals with a Loved One

Sometimes verbalizing goals makes them more real. Sharing your situation can also build camaraderie and support. If you think that sharing your goals with a friend or family member will help you be more excited about the plan and stick with it better, then by all means, tell them what you're doing and why.

You may even inspire the person you tell. If he has acid reflux, he may want to follow in your habit-changing footsteps, or if she's wanting to embark on a different type of diet (say, low fat or lower carb), you may inspire her to do that as well. Perhaps you can both embark on your new diets the same week and check in on each other. Whether it's pure support or a little healthy competition, you may find that working with someone helps you.

Other people are more likely to stick to a goal if they keep it to themselves. Mum's the word for that type of person. He may figure that his diet process will include some relapses, and maybe he won't want to share every one of those bumps in the road with a well-meaning friend or family member who constantly inquires about his progress. Everyone is different, so think about what will work for you and go with that.

Following the Recipes in This Book (And Finding More!)

There are enough recipes in this book to get you started and to keep you satisfied for a couple months, and likely far longer. However, if variety is the spice of life for you and you need to have new recipes every week, modify the recipes in this book or find new ones! The Internet is obviously a great resource. The best resource though, after this book and the Internet, is yourself. Only you know exactly what your trigger foods are — a doctor can only guess. When you know what your trigger foods are, make recipes that avoid them. You'll start doing so subconsciously, most likely. For instance, if garlic bothers you, you'll find that you don't even consider putting garlic in your salsa. You'll modify that recipe without even thinking about it.

Visualizing Yourself Succeeding

You've got your list of goals and you wrote what you want to feel like. That's great. Now, put that paper away and visualize the future. Does the "new you" feel calm and peaceful lying down at night, knowing that reflux won't be a part of your night? Does the "new you" feel better in your clothes and in your skin because you lost weight by following the acid reflux diet?

Do you see yourself strolling through a beer festival content knowing that one beer is your limit and that anything else will trigger reflux, and being totally fine with that? Does the "new you" stop eating when you're full, instead of stuffing yourself and putting dangerous pressure on your lower esophageal sphincter? Does the "new you" just plain feel good? Is that person happier? More patient? That's going to be you! That's what you're working toward. Visualize it, and make it happen!

Going Easy on Yourself

All right, you've written about success, you've visualized yourself successful, and you've followed the steps to be successful. Does that mean you'll meet all your goals all at once? Not necessarily. There will be missteps along the way, and you may relapse. After you start feeling good on a new plan, it's easy to think, "Hey, I've got this! Sweet!" and then start making concessions. Have you ever gone on a diet, lost the weight, and then thought you could go back to your old ways, only to find that the weight came back? That will happen with the acid reflux diet as well, if you stop following it (the reflux will come back).

When your reflux decreases, and your anatomy normalizes and becomes less sensitive, you may find that you can tolerate trigger foods a little better than before. You may be tempted to "push it" by eating those foods again and in bigger quantities. Well, that's okay. You'll learn how far you can push it and how far you can't.

When you suffer those little missteps or relapses (maybe you'll gorge on chocolate at a holiday party, or drink till drunk at a wedding), don't be too hard on yourself. You fell off the wagon, or misunderstood the wagon. Now regroup and climb back on. When you visualize yourself being successful, visualize yourself being understanding, too. Don't waste these valuable experiences: Learn from them. What were the triggers that led you to misstep? Fatigue, lack of planning, lack of motivation? When you know your triggers, you can anticipate them and plan accordingly.

Deciding Whether to Go Cold Turkey or Ease In

Some people change eating habits better when they go cold turkey ("I'm never drinking coffee again!"), while other people do better easing in ("I'm going to cut back from two cups of coffee every day to one cup of coffee every day, to one half a cup a few times a week."). What's important is to find the method that works for you. Some people think that cold turkey is too extreme and that it makes them more likely to throw out the plan. For others, it's the only way. You're the one who knows.

For more information on going cold turkey versus easing in, see Chapter 6.

Giving Yourself Time to Adjust

Whether you go cold turkey or you ease in, allow yourself time for the changes to settle. For instance, you may not have instant relief, or you may not lose weight instantly (and maybe losing weight isn't even your goal). Either way, be patient with the results, and be patient with yourself. You may stumble a little in getting rid of foods that bother you, and it may be tricky to start new habits, especially when it involves getting rid of old habits. Be nice to yourself.

Finding your trigger foods and discovering which amounts of certain foods and beverages you can tolerate may take a while. Don't expect to feel amazing in a day or a week. Just hope to feel considerably better one month after starting your new plan, and maybe you'll feel considerably better at the end of the second month than you felt at the end of the first.

Looking for the Silver Lining

As much as you want positive results, it's surprisingly easy to ignore them. A key to changing eating habits is to celebrate the victories that come along with the change. If three weeks after you start this plan, you generally feel really good, acknowledge that. The positive reinforcement will encourage you to stay on the positive plan. Revisit your goals list and see how many of them you're meeting. Write down how you feel now that your health is improving. For instance, "I feel well rested because I'm sleeping better. I fit in my clothes better because I'm eating less and losing weight. I feel more balanced, because I'm getting my reflux under control."

Chapter 19

Ten Changes You Can Make in the Kitchen

In This Chapter

▶ Considering cooking methods

▶ Reducing certain ingredients

▶ Substituting some ingredients for others

Following a reflux-friendly diet isn't draconian or iron clad. It involves looking at foods and habits in new ways and making substitutions when necessary. The ten tips in this chapter will make the changes easier, and before you know it you'll be following these guidelines without even thinking about them.

You won't identify yourself as being on an acid-reflux diet — you'll just be someone who does some things a little differently than you used to, and who feels better than ever.

Sautéing

Sometimes, frying food makes it the most delicious it can be. But frying also tends to make food the fattiest it can be. Excess fat is terrible for reflux sufferers. If you get worse reflux when you eat fried foods, then either give up fried foods entirely or eat them in tiny amounts and infrequently. Unless you're used to eating, say, fried chicken every day of your life, you probably won't feel like there's a gaping hole when you make a reduction.

Another reason to reduce fried food: Many restaurants reheat previously used oil to fry food. Reheated oils have been found to produce toxins that, when consumed, have been found to increase the risk of several diseases, including cancer.

Start sautéing food instead of frying it, and you'll still be able to enjoy most of the same ingredients, just in a different way. Sautéing is easier, safer, and will leave less grease on your stove and counter.

All you need is a burner, a frying pan (any size), and a little oil. Some oils are healthier than others — in general, olive oil is the best choice, but the most common type of oil for sautéing is vegetable oil. In small portions, any type of oil (including vegetable oil) is fine, but because olive oil has more health benefits and is lower in calories, give it a try instead. Plus, it's a little thinner than vegetable oil, so you don't need as much to coat a pan.

Turn your burner on medium heat, and let the pan get hot — it'll take at least a minute. When the pan is hot, add enough oil to very thinly coat the bottom of the pan (anywhere from 1 to 3 tablespoons, depending on how much food you'll be cooking). Add salt and pepper and any other seasoning you like. Wait a minute or two until the oil is hot. Then add the food you want to sauté. You'll know the pan and oil are hot enough if the food sizzles when it hits the pan. Cook until golden brown, turning the food as necessary.

Baking, Broiling, or Roasting

Baking, broiling, and roasting take longer than frying, but these methods require much less fat (which means less reflux) and can lock in a unique flavor that frying and even sautéing can't achieve.

Broiling and roasting, in particular, make ingredients taste even more like themselves. Cover whatever you're cooking with foil or a lid and many foods will become incredibly moist. Root vegetables are especially successful roasted, and many meats taste their best cooked in this fashion, too.

Steaming

Steaming is one of the lowest-fat ways of cooking. It can work well for vegetables, but it can also make them mushy and lifeless if you steam them too long.

To steam, put a soup pot or saucepan on top of a burner. Pour water in the pan or pot, turn on the burner, and let the water come to a boil. Add a steamer basket to the top of the pan or pot. Add your vegetables to the basket.

When the color of the vegetables becomes a little more vivid than when they were raw, and when the vegetables have a little give, remove the basket from the steam. If you like your vegetables to have a nice crunch or to be chewy, cook for less time.

The mushier you want your vegetables, the longer you should steam them. However, when the color starts to look brownish or grayish, it's definitely time to take the vegetables off the steam.

You can season before, during, or after steaming.

Boiling

Boiling can be a good cooking option that can turn bad quickly. Over-boiling is probably the sole reason why generations of Americans hate Brussels sprouts — Brussels sprouts (and many other vegetables) taste much better roasted or sautéed than boiled. However, if you *do* boil them, they still can taste good as long as you don't boil them beyond recognition. No vegetable should be mushy or pasty.

Vegetables are at their best when they reach their most vivid color. After that, they may have been in the water too long.

Always bring the water to a boil before putting the food in, as opposed to letting the food come to a boil along with the water. Remove from the water, drain, and season.

Less Is More

Portion control is huge (ironic) when it comes to reducing acid reflux. Some main tips to remember for getting rid of acid reflux, or reducing it, are to eat the right foods, avoid the wrong foods, and eat the right portions. Within reason, the smaller the meal, the better. You want to reduce pressure on the lower-esophageal sphincter (LES). Putting too much food in your system increases pressure beyond what that poor LES can take, and you suffer for it later.

The human stomach is only about the size of an adult's cupped hands. Yes, it stretches out, but if you're stretching it out too much and too often, chances are, the consequence will be acid reflux.

Avoiding Trigger Ingredients

Everyone has different trigger ingredients, but there are themes for sure. For instance, citrus, alcohol, and garlic are popular culprits. Find out what your triggers are, and avoid them. For a list of potential problem foods, see Chapter 4. To take a trigger test/elimination experiment, follow the guidelines in Chapter 6.

Adding Soothing Ingredients

Isn't it great that there are foods that are actually good for getting rid of reflux? See, it's not just about avoidance! Try to add neutral, non-bothersome foods to your daily life. For a list of soothing ingredients, see Chapter 6.

Drinking Wisely

So, you start sautéing instead of frying, you cut out trigger foods, and you increase soothing foods in your diet. You lose weight, exercise, and change your sleep position. You even quit smoking! All that has a great chance of working. However, if you wash the right foods in the right amounts down with the wrong beverage, you may continue to suffer from reflux.

 Avoid soda and carbonated water, avoid juice unless you water it down dramatically, avoid caffeinated beverages, go easy on alcohol, and when in doubt, drink water. If you get sick of water, add fruit or herbs to give it a little flavor. Drinking lots of water is great for your health, and it also helps thin out the reflux that may come up — the thinner it is, the easier it will be to get out of your throat, and the less potent that fiery mess will be.

For reflux-friendly drink recipes, see Chapter 13.

Reduce Meat Portions

The fattier the meat, the worse it is for acid reflux. The slower the fatty meat leaves your stomach, the worse it is for acid reflux. Keeping portions small is important for getting rid of reflux, and this is particularly true for meats. Minimize red meat and go for poultry or fish instead.

Reducing or Substituting Fat

Earlier in this chapter, we provide tips for cooking with less fat. However, you can also reduce fat by using less of it in your recipes. For baked goods, applesauce can be a great replacement for fat (you can also do half–traditional fat and half-applesauce). You can replace full-fat butter with reduced-fat butter and/or eat smaller quantities of it. Same with all dairy products.

Chapter 20

Ten Myths about Acid Reflux

In This Chapter

▶ Dispelling common myths about reflux

▶ Getting to the truth about the condition

*I*f you've been vocal about your acid reflux, you've heard it all by now. Loved ones and complete strangers have probably offered advice and information. Some of it may be true, and some of it may be myth. How do you know for sure? You can research on the Internet, but there are plenty of myths there, too.

In this chapter, we set the record straight on acid reflux, debunking some common myths about the disease. So, next time you get "helpful" advice from someone, whether your uncle, sister, colleague, or spouse, turn to this book, and this chapter in particular, to get the truth.

The Heart Is What Causes Heartburn

"Heartburn." What a misnomer. Heartburn has nothing to do with the heart, except that the chest (which, of course, houses the heart) is the general location where people with acid reflux feel discomfort. But the condition of the heart has nothing to do with whether someone suffers from acid reflux.

Acid Reflux Kills Bad Breath

Some people think that the acid that shoots up your esophagus kills bad-breath germs. Nope. Acid reflux can make the condition worse.

Heartburn Is No Big Deal

Heartburn is common. More than 60 million Americans experience heartburn or other reflux symptoms at least once a month. About 30 percent of Americans have chronic acid reflux or gastroesophageal reflux disease (GERD). That's a lot of people.

But just because the condition is common doesn't mean we shouldn't worry about it. Acid reflux should be taken seriously. First, it's uncomfortable, if not outright painful. It can cause missed sleep, make you cranky, and lead to GERD. And what can GERD lead to? Barrett's esophagus. And what can Barrett's esophagus lead to? That's right, esophageal cancer.

Acid reflux is no big deal if you have it a couple times a year. The more often you get it though, and the more severe it is, the more you need to worry about it. So, is acid reflux a big deal? Yes, it is.

Prescription Drugs for Acid Reflux Hurt the Digestion Process

Some drugs for heartburn and reflux reduce the amount of acid people have in their stomachs. Acid is a vital part of the digestion process, which is why some people wonder if taking medicine that reduces acid will hurt digestion. No fear, though: The stomach keeps producing enough acid for digestion.

Gastroesophageal Reflux Disease Always Leads to Cancer

GERD can lead to Barrett's esophagus, and Barrett's esophagus can lead to esophageal cancer. The keyword is *can*. If you have GERD, you're not destined to develop Barrett's esophagus, and if you have Barrett's esophagus, you're not destined to develop cancer.

Only between 5 percent and 10 percent of GERD patients develop Barrett's esophagus. And only 0.5 percent of Barrett's esophagus patients develop esophageal cancer per year.

For more information on GERD and Barrett's esophagus, turn to Chapter 3.

Only Unhealthy People Get Acid Reflux

You have to be obese, have muscle atrophy and cataracts, and be an alcoholic to get acid reflux, right? Nope!

Otherwise completely healthy people can get acid reflux regularly. Now, people who are unhealthy in certain ways (smokers, frequent drinkers, and so on) are more likely to develop acid reflux, but totally healthy people can develop it, too. Athletes get it, yoga teachers get it, nutritionists get it.

If you have certain habits, you can get acid reflux, even if you're at a perfect weight, eat well, and exercise regularly.

Heartburn Is Just Part of the Aging Process

Not so. Yes, the digestion process does slow down as we age, and that slow-down can make someone a little more likely to suffer from acid reflux, but that doesn't mean that seniors are destined to get it. As at any other age, diet and lifestyle changes can minimize your chances of developing reflux. Acid reflux is not inevitable just because you're a certain age.

Over-the-Counter Antacids Aren't Real Medicine

Over-the-counter acid-reflux pills don't require a prescription, but they're still a medicine, and they do have side effects. Some people pop antacids like candy, but no one should do that. Read the instructions for use and follow them. Antacids are some of the most common and best-selling drugs in the world because they provide comfort in many cases. However, they do *not* cure acid reflux and abuse of them can cause side effects like the following:

- Loss of appetite
- Excessive tiredness
- Weakness
- Diarrhea
- Muscle pain
- Swelling

- ✔ Kidney stones
- ✔ Liver damage
- ✔ Senility
- ✔ Memory loss
- ✔ Dementia

If you fear you're ingesting too many antacids, contact your doctor immediately for consultation, and be honest about exactly what kind of antacid you take, how many antacids you're taking, and when.

It Doesn't Matter What Side of Your Body You Sleep On

Some people swear that it doesn't matter which side they sleep on. However, if you're prone to acid reflux at night, you should lie on your left side. The digestive tract runs in such a way that lying on your left side makes acid reflux much less likely. See, the stomach is located to the left of the esophagus, which makes it hard for acid to flow out of the stomach and into the esophagus. Lie on your right side and you're more likely to get acid reflux.

In this case, right is wrong.

Drinking Decaffeinated Coffee Won't Aggravate Your Acid Reflux

Not so. It's the oil in the beans (caffeinated or non) that can cause reflux. So, whether caffeinated or decaf or half-caff, that cup of coffee may cause you problems. Now, if you aren't bothered by any type of coffee, you're okay here and can drink caffeinated or decaf, whatever your preference.

Chapter 21

Ten Benefits of Getting Rid of Acid Reflux

In This Chapter

▶ Understanding why the fight against reflux matters

▶ Seeing how reflux affects your life

▶ Imagining a life post-reflux

A s you know, getting rid of acid reflux has many benefits. Some are directly related to the elimination of reflux symptoms, while others are secondary benefits that stem from reflux-reduction efforts (for instance, you may lose weight). Some benefits impact physical health, while others impact quality of life. All are important. We highlight some of these benefits in this chapter, in case you need a refresher on why you're making all those lifestyle changes.

A Good Night's Sleep

The most common complaint from reflux patients pertains to how the reflux messes with sleep. Whether it's preventing you from falling asleep, waking you up, or just making you uncomfortable, reflux can be the nemesis of a good night's sleep.

The fact that most people eat their largest meal of the day at dinner is just one factor that plays a part here. Lying down is another. When you lie down, this position removes gravity from the battle and makes it easier for your stomach's contents to enter your esophagus. Whatever the cause, acid reflux can turn a night's rest into a nightmare.

Studies have routinely shown a link between insufficient sleep and health problems such as heart disease, heart attacks, diabetes, and obesity. Proper rest also plays a critical role in pain management, especially for people dealing with chronic or acute pain. Sleep can also influence mood, weight, concentration, memory, and even your sex life.

With sleep playing such a vital role in so many aspects of life, it's clear that eliminating reflux and improving sleep is one of those gifts that keeps on giving.

Better Overall Health

One of the most common ways doctors advocate treating reflux is through dietary changes. Fortunately, many of the dietary changes recommended for the treatment of reflux will also have a positive affect on your overall health. One of the most notorious dietary culprits associated with reflux is high-fat food. Next to smoking, high-fat diets are the most lethal personal habit, contributing to an estimated 300,000 deaths annually in the United States alone. High-fat diets have been linked to obesity, heart disease, stroke, cancer, high blood pressure, and diabetes. Clearly, cutting a little (or a lot of) fatty or fried food from your diet isn't such a bad idea.

When you have reflux, doctors also recommend minimizing alcohol intake and quitting tobacco as well. Although drinking alcohol in moderation is usually harmless, chronic alcohol use is linked to cancer, heart disease, cirrhosis, dementia, depression, seizures, and high blood pressure. Likewise, smoking has been connected with a variety of health problems, many of which can be fatal. It may not seem like fun, but reducing alcohol intake and quitting smoking as part of your reflux attack plan will reduce your risk for serious conditions like heart disease and cancer, while helping put a cap on your reflux as well.

Bottom line: When you make the lifestyle changes that your doctor recommends to reduce your reflux symptoms, your body will benefit in all kinds of other ways, too!

Goodbye Heartburn

An even more important benefit for many patients is the elimination of the chronic pain associated with reflux. As anyone who has dealt with chronic pain can attest, there's nothing fun about daily discomfort. For many people with acid reflux, chronic pain becomes a part of the package. Often it's associated with heartburn, but it can also result from other complications associated with reflux, such as a sore throat or an esophageal stricture. Regardless of the cause, chronic pain can affect everything from your physical ability to overall happiness.

Imagine what a relief it would be not to have to worry about facing hours of discomfort every time you eat a meal. Imagine not having to worry about having your reflux medication or antacids with you at all times. Eliminating chronic pain and discomfort associated with reflux from your daily life is well worth the effort and cost involved in treating reflux.

A Clearer Mind

Getting rid of reflux can also have a positive impact on cognitive abilities. The interrupted sleep and pain associated with reflux can have a profound impact on a person's ability to concentrate and think clearly. Dealing with reflux on a regular basis could affect grades, relationships, or job performance. Plus, dealing with the hallmarks of acid reflux (such as chronic heartburn, loss of sleep, and poor diet) also improve mental abilities.

Study after study has shown how dramatic an impact sleep has on mental function. Driving without sufficient sleep can be as dangerous as driving drunk. Add the constant discomfort and distraction caused by scorching heartburn, and it's clear how significantly acid reflux can affect your ability to function and think.

A Brighter Disposition

It's not just mental capabilities that can be affected; it's also your attitude and emotions. Even the brightest disposition can be worn down by years of chronic heartburn, insufficient sleep, and other complications associated with reflux. It's hard to be happy and enjoy life when you're exhausted from battling reflux.

And it's not only *your* mood that will be affected, it's the moods of all those around you. As anyone who has ever dealt with a teenager knows, tired and cranky people can bring everyone down. Reflux can make you moody, hostile, or even depressed. You can hardly be blamed for being a little grouchy after a few hours of really bad heartburn or a night of restless tossing and turning. But think about how your poor family and coworkers must feel when you're moody or depressed on a regular basis. In this case, getting rid of your reflux can have benefits for those around you as well.

Even if you're one of the lucky ones whose reflux doesn't altar your mood, imagine how much happier you'd be if you didn't have to deal with reflux at all. When you take into account all the time, money, discomfort, and trouble it takes to deal with serious cases of acid reflux it's understandable that reflux can be a mood killer.

Less Stress

Having to carry the burden of acid reflux on a daily basis can be draining. For many people, reflux has an impact on their day-to-day activities. It doesn't just impact what they eat or drink; it also affects what they can and can't do. It's common for patients to tell their doctors stories about how reflux prevents them from going about their daily business. All of this worrying equals stress.

Whether it's not wanting to go out for a bite to eat with friends, or worrying every time you go to run errands that reflux will stop you in your tracks, getting reflux under control can be the first step in taking back your life and decreasing your stress levels.

Decreasing stress literally changes the chemistry of your body. By having fewer things to worry about, your body will produce fewer stress hormones, such as cortisol. With fewer of these hormones, your heart rate will be healthier, you'll digest food better, feel calmer and happier, and be less prone to illness.

Fewer Doctor Visits

Many of the lifestyle changes required to manage acid reflux are beneficial for overall health, as we mention earlier. A well-balanced diet will ensure that your body is getting all the nutrients and energy it needs, which may give you fewer reasons to visit the doctor.

Tame the Flame, Stop the Inflammation

If you have asthma, chronic cough, and chronic sore throat, eliminating reflux is particularly important. A direct link between asthma and acid reflux hasn't been proven, but evidence suggests that reflux can trigger or worsen asthma attacks. It's also important to note that 75 percent of people with asthma reported suffering from at least occasional acid reflux. Studies show that reducing or eliminating reflux can lead to a reduction of asthma attacks, as well as the severity of those attacks. As it turns out, treating your reflux may be one of the keys to helping you manage asthma as well.

It's no surprise that chronic coughs and chronic sore throats are often associated with acid reflux. When you have corrosive stomach acid firing into your esophagus and throat, it's inevitable that there will be at least a little damage and pain involved.

People who complain of chronic coughs or sore throats often are diagnosed with acid reflux. Even in situations where reflux isn't the main culprit, it doesn't take a stretch of the imagination to realize that splashing stomach acid onto an already irritated or inflamed throat and lungs would make things worse. If reflux is the reason for your inflammation and discomfort, reducing or eliminating reflux can mean saying bye-bye to your cough or sore throat.

Imagine being able to go to the movies without having to worry that a coughing spell will ruin the experience. Contemplate eating a meal or having a drink without worrying about how much swallowing is going to hurt. When your reflux is under control, you won't have to imagine it — you'll be living it!

Reduced Risk for Cancer

By eliminating reflux, you can significantly reduce your risk for developing serious medical conditions. One of the most serious conditions associated with acid reflux and gastroesophageal reflux disease (GERD) is Barrett's esophagus. Barrett's esophagus is a condition in which the tissue lining the esophagus is altered for the worse. Frequent reflux means the esophagus is constantly having to repair itself from damage. The more your esophagus has to repair itself, the more opportunities your cells have to develop abnormally.

As if Barrett's weren't scary enough on its own, it can occasionally lead to esophageal cancer. In fact, your risk for developing esophageal cancer goes up every year you have Barrett's. And esophageal cancer is nothing to joke about. Patients who don't have surgical treatment for their cancer have only a 10 percent five-year survival rate. Even for those who get surgery, the five-year survival rate is between 5 percent and 30 percent. Those who catch it in the early stages have the best chances for survival. This means reducing or eliminating your reflux won't only affect the quality of your life and overall health, but it may actually end up saving your life.

Show Me the Money!

The final place you'll see a benefit of an acid-free life is in your wallet. If you've been battling acid reflux for very long, you know that the battle is rarely free. Whether your reflux is minor enough to be treated with the occasional antacid, or you have to shell out for prescription meds on a monthly basis, there's a cost to fighting reflux.

Many reflux sufferers buy copious amounts of antacids, and that adds up. Other sufferers make frequent visits to the doctor, and those co-pays add up. And if you require long-term medication to help manage your heartburn, you may resent that expense. Medications can do a number on your wallet. However, the cost of medication is a small price to pay compared to the cost of surgery — surgery can be astronomically expensive, and it may cause you to miss work, which means losing more money.

Besides the huge health benefits of beating reflux, look to your wallet for inspiration in your battle against acid reflux and GERD.

For some people, medication is part or all of what helps them beat acid reflux, and they need it lifelong. For others, however, the medication is a stopgap and they can get off the medication eventually. The people who get to stop taking medication not only have a more convenient life, but also save money.

Appendix

Metric Conversion Guide

· ·

Note: The recipes in this book weren't developed or tested using metric measurements. There may be some variation in quality when converting to metric units.

Common Abbreviations

Abbreviation(s)	What It Stands For
cm	Centimeter
C., c.	Cup
G, g	Gram
kg	Kilogram
L, l	Liter
lb.	Pound
mL, ml	Milliliter
oz.	Ounce
pt.	Pint
t., tsp.	Teaspoon
T., Tb., Tbsp.	Tablespoon

Volume

U.S. Units	Canadian Metric	Australian Metric
¼ teaspoon	1 milliliter	1 milliliter
½ teaspoon	2 milliliters	2 milliliters
1 teaspoon	5 milliliters	5 milliliters
1 tablespoon	15 milliliters	20 milliliters

(continued)

Volume *(continued)*

U.S. Units	Canadian Metric	Australian Metric
¼ cup	50 milliliters	60 milliliters
⅓ cup	75 milliliters	80 milliliters
½ cup	125 milliliters	125 milliliters
⅔ cup	150 milliliters	170 milliliters
¾ cup	175 milliliters	190 milliliters
1 cup	250 milliliters	250 milliliters
1 quart	1 liter	1 liter
1½ quarts	1.5 liters	1.5 liters
2 quarts	2 liters	2 liters
2½ quarts	2.5 liters	2.5 liters
3 quarts	3 liters	3 liters
4 quarts (1 gallon)	4 liters	4 liters

Weight

U.S. Units	Canadian Metric	Australian Metric
1 ounce	30 grams	30 grams
2 ounces	55 grams	60 grams
3 ounces	85 grams	90 grams
4 ounces (¼ pound)	115 grams	125 grams
8 ounces (½ pound)	225 grams	225 grams
16 ounces (1 pound)	455 grams	500 grams (½ kilogram)

Length

Inches	Centimeters
0.5	1.5
1	2.5
2	5.0
3	7.5

Inches	Centimeters
4	10.0
5	12.5
6	15.0
7	17.5
8	20.5
9	23.0
10	25.5
11	28.0
12	30.5

Temperature (Degrees)

Fahrenheit	Celsius
32	0
212	100
250	120
275	140
300	150
325	160
350	180
375	190
400	200
425	220
450	230
475	240
500	260

Index

• C •

• H •

• *M* •

• *N* •

• V •

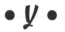

Notes

About the Authors

Patricia Raymond, MD, FACG: Dr. Raymond is a practicing gastroenterologist in Virginia and Assistant Professor of Clinical Internal Medicine at Eastern Virginia Medical School. She is one of the most respected voices in patient education regarding digestive health, including acid reflux. Her articles and books help people function better south of the mouth. All this with a dose of levity — "belly laughter," if you will.

Dr. Raymond's medical music parodies were honored with a nomination for the WEGO Hilarious Health Activist Award in 2012 and 2013. She is a fellow with the American College of Gastroenterology and is an affiliate member of the Society of Gastroenterology Nurses and Associates. Dr. Raymond is a frequent keynote speaker at regional and national healthcare conferences, where she discusses digestive health and patient empowerment.

Michelle Beaver: Michelle has served as editor-in-chief or associate editor for magazines that serve surgeons, endoscopic nurses, nephrologists, and primary-care physicians. She has written about digestive health for eight years. Michelle has taught journalism at Arizona State University's Walter Cronkite School of Journalism and Mass Communication, and Scottsdale Community College, where she serves on the Journalism Department advisory board. She has reported for the Associated Press and publications such as the *Oakland Tribune* and the *San Jose Mercury News*. Michelle volunteers weekly with Boys Hope Girls Hope and enjoys spending time with her friends, family, and cats.

Authors' Acknowledgments

We're indebted to several people in the writing of this book, most of all dietitian extraordinaire, Sonnet Bingham Aguirre. Despite working full-time in a hospital, teaching at a university, and being pregnant, Sonnet provided many of the wonderful recipes in this book and was kindly available for our many questions. Her experiences and research appear throughout this book.

Many thanks to journalist Steven Leslie for his help with research and special projects. We're grateful for his ability and helpfulness. We also appreciate the talented *For Dummies* team at John Wiley & Sons, most of all our acquisitions editor, Tracy Boggier, and project editor, Elizabeth Kuball. Both were amiable and knowledgeable through our entire process. We're also grateful for our agent, Matt Wagner.

Michelle Beaver would like to thank Keith Chartier for his help with everything, always, and the fine people at Lux coffee shop in Phoenix for their encouragement.

Patricia Raymond would like to acknowledge the "stamina and sheer grit" of her colleague, Ms. Beaver, and Michelle would like to respond by saying, "Patricia, I've enjoyed working with you on various projects for five years and I look up to you. You're a wonderful doctor, writer, and educator." On that note, the authors would like to thank you, the reader, for making it through these lengthy acknowledgments.

Publisher's Acknowledgments

Senior Acquisitions Editor: Tracy Boggier

Project Editor: Elizabeth Kuball

Copy Editor: Elizabeth Kuball

Technical Editor: Rachel Nix

Recipe Tester: Emily Nolan

Nutrition Analyst: Patricia Santelli

Project Coordinator: Patrick Redmond

Photographer: T. J. Hines

Cover Image: ©iStockphoto.com/ GerryWilsonStudios

Apple & Mac

iPad For Dummies,
6th Edition
978-1-118-72306-7

iPhone For Dummies,
7th Edition
978-1-118-69083-3

Macs All-in-One
For Dummies, 4th Edition
978-1-118-82210-4

OS X Mavericks
For Dummies
978-1-118-69188-5

Blogging & Social Media

Facebook For Dummies,
5th Edition
978-1-118-63312-0

Social Media Engagement
For Dummies
978-1-118-53019-1

WordPress For Dummies,
6th Edition
978-1-118-79161-5

Business

Stock Investing
For Dummies, 4th Edition
978-1-118-37678-2

Investing For Dummies,
6th Edition
978-0-470-90545-6

Personal Finance
For Dummies, 7th Edition
978-1-118-11785-9

QuickBooks 2014
For Dummies
978-1-118-72005-9

Small Business Marketing
Kit For Dummies,
3rd Edition
978-1-118-31183-7

Careers

Job Interviews
For Dummies, 4th Edition
978-1-118-11290-8

Job Searching with Social
Media For Dummies,
2nd Edition
978-1-118-67856-5

Personal Branding
For Dummies
978-1-118-11792-7

Resumes For Dummies,
6th Edition
978-0-470-87361-8

Starting an Etsy Business
For Dummies, 2nd Edition
978-1-118-59024-9

Diet & Nutrition

Belly Fat Diet For Dummies
978-1-118-34585-6

Mediterranean Diet
For Dummies
978-1-118-71525-3

Nutrition For Dummies,
5th Edition
978-0-470-93231-5

Digital Photography

Digital SLR Photography
All-in-One For Dummies,
2nd Edition
978-1-118-59082-9

Digital SLR Video &
Filmmaking For Dummies
978-1-118-36598-4

Photoshop Elements 12
For Dummies
978-1-118-72714-0

Gardening

Herb Gardening
For Dummies, 2nd Edition
978-0-470-61778-6

Gardening with Free-Range
Chickens For Dummies
978-1-118-54754-0

Health

Boosting Your Immunity
For Dummies
978-1-118-40200-9

Diabetes For Dummies,
4th Edition
978-1-118-29447-5

Living Paleo For Dummies
978-1-118-29405-5

Big Data

Big Data For Dummies
978-1-118-50422-2

Data Visualization
For Dummies
978-1-118-50289-1

Hadoop For Dummies
978-1-118-60755-8

Language &
Foreign Language

500 Spanish Verbs
For Dummies
978-1-118-02382-2

English Grammar
For Dummies, 2nd Edition
978-0-470-54664-2

French All-in-One
For Dummies
978-1-118-22815-9

German Essentials
For Dummies
978-1-118-18422-6

Italian For Dummies,
2nd Edition
978-1-118-00465-4

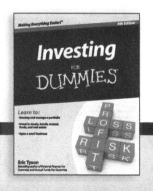
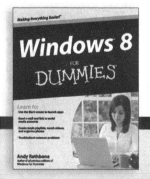
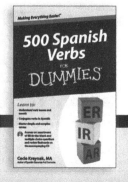
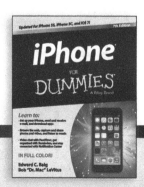

Math & Science

Algebra I For Dummies,
2nd Edition
978-0-470-55964-2

Anatomy and Physiology
For Dummies, 2nd Edition
978-0-470-92326-9

Astronomy For Dummies,
3rd Edition
978-1-118-37697-3

Biology For Dummies,
2nd Edition
978-0-470-59875-7

Chemistry For Dummies,
2nd Edition
978-1-118-00730-3

1001 Algebra II Practice
Problems For Dummies
978-1-118-44662-1

Microsoft Office

Excel 2013 For Dummies
978-1-118-51012-4

Office 2013 All-in-One
For Dummies
978-1-118-51636-2

PowerPoint 2013
For Dummies
978-1-118-50253-2

Word 2013 For Dummies
978-1-118-49123-2

Music

Blues Harmonica
For Dummies
978-1-118-25269-7

Guitar For Dummies,
3rd Edition
978-1-118-11554-1

iPod & iTunes
For Dummies, 10th Edition
978-1-118-50864-0

Programming

Beginning Programming
with C For Dummies
978-1-118-73763-7

Excel VBA Programming
For Dummies, 3rd Edition
978-1-118-49037-2

Java For Dummies,
6th Edition
978-1-118-40780-6

Religion & Inspiration

The Bible For Dummies
978-0-7645-5296-0

Buddhism For Dummies,
2nd Edition
978-1-118-02379-2

Catholicism For Dummies,
2nd Edition
978-1-118-07778-8

Self-Help & Relationships

Beating Sugar Addiction
For Dummies
978-1-118-54645-1

Meditation For Dummies,
3rd Edition
978-1-118-29144-3

Seniors

Laptops For Seniors
For Dummies, 3rd Edition
978-1-118-71105-7

Computers For Seniors
For Dummies, 3rd Edition
978-1-118-11553-4

iPad For Seniors
For Dummies, 6th Edition
978-1-118-72826-0

Social Security
For Dummies
978-1-118-20573-0

Smartphones & Tablets

Android Phones
For Dummies, 2nd Edition
978-1-118-72030-1

Nexus Tablets
For Dummies
978-1-118-77243-0

Samsung Galaxy S 4
For Dummies
978-1-118-64222-1

Samsung Galaxy Tabs
For Dummies
978-1-118-77294-2

Test Prep

ACT For Dummies,
5th Edition
978-1-118-01259-8

ASVAB For Dummies,
3rd Edition
978-0-470-63760-9

GRE For Dummies,
7th Edition
978-0-470-88921-3

Officer Candidate Tests
For Dummies
978-0-470-59876-4

Physician's Assistant Exam
For Dummies
978-1-118-11556-5

Series 7 Exam For Dummies
978-0-470-09932-2

Windows 8

Windows 8.1 All-in-One
For Dummies
978-1-118-82087-2

Windows 8.1 For Dummies
978-1-118-82121-3

Windows 8.1 For Dummies
Book + DVD Bundle
978-1-118-82107-7

Available in print and e-book formats.

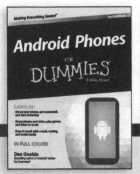
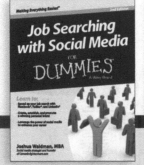
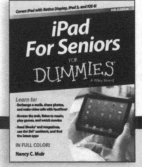
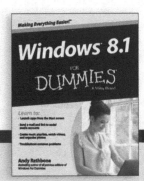

Available wherever books are sold. **For more information or to order direct visit www.dummies.com**

Take Dummies with you everywhere you go!

Whether you are excited about e-books, want more from the web, must have your mobile apps, or are swept up in social media, Dummies makes everything easier.

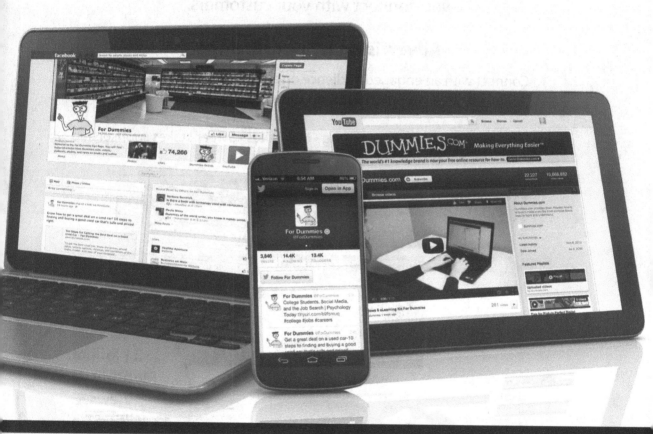

Leverage the Power

For Dummies is the global leader in the reference category and one of the most trusted and highly regarded brands in the world. No longer just focused on books, customers now have access to the For Dummies content they need in the format they want. Let us help you develop a solution that will fit your brand and help you connect with your customers.

Advertising & Sponsorships

Connect with an engaged audience on a powerful multimedia site, and position your message alongside expert how-to content.

Targeted ads • Video • Email marketing • Microsites • Sweepstakes sponsorship

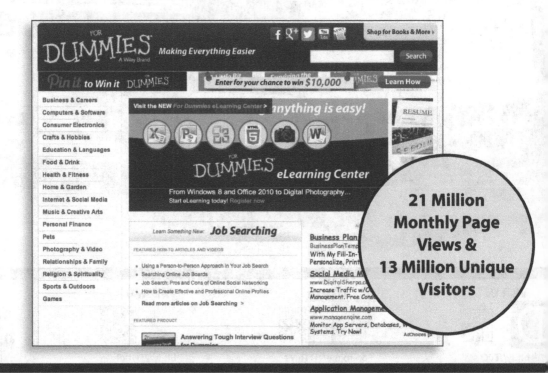

# of For Dummies

Custom Publishing

Reach a global audience in any language by creating a solution that will differentiate you from competitors, amplify your message, and encourage customers to make a buying decision.

Apps • Books • eBooks • Video • Audio • Webinars

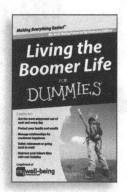 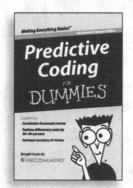 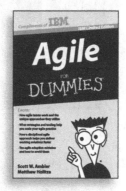 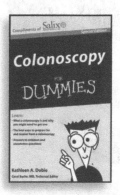

Brand Licensing & Content

Leverage the strength of the world's most popular reference brand to reach new audiences and channels of distribution.

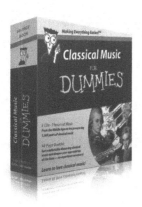 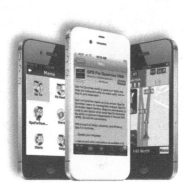 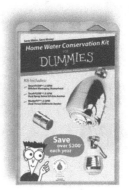 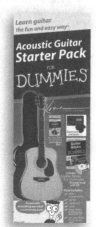

For more information, visit www.Dummies.com/biz

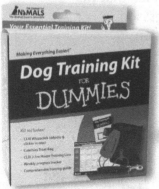
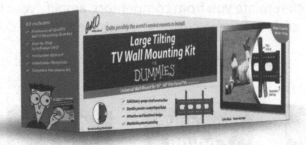
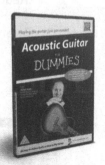
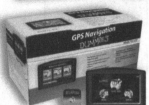
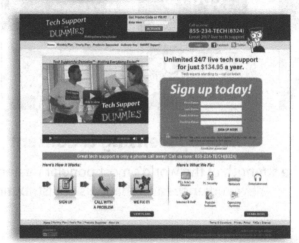
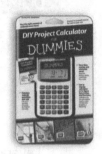
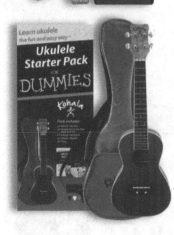
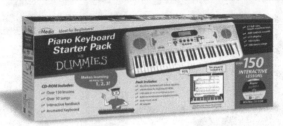
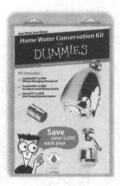